Peripheral Neuropathy
& Neuropathic Pain

Into the Light

Written by one of the world's leading experts
Gérard Said MD FRCP

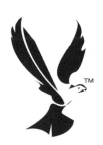

i

tfm Publishing Limited, Castle Hill Barns, Harley, Shrewsbury, SY5 6LX, UK
Tel: +44 (0)1952 510061; Fax: +44 (0)1952 510192
E-mail: info@tfmpublishing.com
Web site: www.tfmpublishing.com

Editing, design & typesetting: Nikki Bramhill BSc Hons Dip Law
First edition: © 2015
Front cover image: © 2014 Andy Keen; web site: www.aurorabasecamp.com

Paperback	ISBN: 978-1-908986-99-3
E-book editions:	2015
ePub	ISBN: 978-1-910079-00-3
Mobi	ISBN: 978-1-910079-01-0
Web pdf	ISBN: 978-1-910079-02-7

Printed by Gutenberg Press Ltd., Gudja Road, Tarxien, PLA 19, Malta

Contents

Foreword

"The pathway from initial presentation to a GP, to hospital consultation, investigations, feedback and review was protracted for a substantial portion of this predominantly elderly, disabled and distressed population, the vast majority of whom reported neuropathic pain symptoms. Dissatisfaction with the management of peripheral neuropathy and pain was the norm and this was associated with diagnostic delay...."

Illness and treatment experience of patients with peripheral neuropathy and neuropathic pain. CK Booker and A Keen, 2004

Whilst it is now true that over the last decade diagnostic and treatment pathways in relation to pain have improved significantly, the diagnosis and treatment of neuropathies generally have perhaps not yet entirely kept pace. It is hoped that this small but valuable book will help to redress this imbalance and add to the slowly growing momentum for change. The peripheral neuropathies may well be a challenging study but, with the guidance of a skilled and experienced tutor such as Professor Gérard Said, it can be readily seen that such a 'challenging study' can be both fascinating and also extremely rewarding.

Nothing can equal the obvious relief when a patient with peripheral neuropathy realises that the health professional they are facing knows even a little about their condition and just some of the ways in which it may affect them as an individual.

The lack of a long-term prognosis, serious disruption of normal social life, pain, depression and anxiety — all may contribute to affect the well-being of people affected by peripheral neuropathy. For a significant number of such people it is not always possible to discover the underlying cause of their problem (the so-called idiopathic/cryptogenic neuropathies). As well as the difficulties due to their primary symptoms, not having a definitive diagnosis may also be of great concern to many individuals.

Again, we feel that this particular publication will be welcomed by all health professionals who come into contact with patients suffering with peripheral neuropathy, and also by patients who may wish to discover more about their own condition.

The production of this book is entirely due to the impetus and support provided by the members of a UK-based charitable organisation — The Neuropathy Trust (1998 - 2014) — and the kindness and hard work of French neurologist, Professor Gérard Said, one of the world's leading experts on peripheral neuropathy. Not only is it a good example of 'Entente Cordiale' but it also demonstrates the very positive results possible when doctors and patients work together in harmony.

Although The Neuropathy Trust has now come to the end of its intended journey, it was felt that the educational side of the Trust's work should continue. Thus, a new organisation has been formed to fulfil this purpose — NeuINsight (www.neuinsight.com). NeuInsight will continue on this important mission and has plans to expand upon the existing educational resources.

Carpe diem.

Andrew Keen
CEO and Founder, The Neuropathy Trust

Acknowledgements

As in many human endeavours it is rare that any successful project is due to any one person alone. The same is true of this particular book, *Peripheral Neuropathy & Neuropathic Pain — Into the Light.*

The first vote of thanks should properly go to all of those people who have supported The Neuropathy Trust from its inception in 1998, through to its closure in 2014. Of these kind people, Mrs Angela Geen, Mrs Diane Vaughan and Mr Douglas Stephenson deserve particular mention for all of their voluntary efforts.

Mrs Belinda Rimmer, her husband Paul and son Edward also deserve a special mention for their constancy and kindness in their fundraising ventures over the last ten years.

Our thanks also go to all of the medical advisors of The Neuropathy Trust, particularly to Dr. Simon J. Ellis, Consultant Neurologist from the University Hospital of North Staffordshire who, apart from assisting the Trust on many occasions, has provided advice and guidance on this book project also.

The main vote of thanks, of course, goes to Professor Gérard Said who has worked so hard — against a very tight deadline — to write this book for us. Gérard is not only a very accomplished neurologist, specialising in peripheral neuropathy, but he has endeared himself to us all by allowing The Neuropathy Trust free access to all professional meetings of the European Neurological Society (an organisation of which he is co-founder). Such generous access has allowed us to keep abreast of all scientific developments and pass the information on to our members via our *Relay* magazine. This 'open access' to a patient group, in the days when it was not particularly fashionable to permit such transparency, is a measure of his calibre — both as a doctor and as a humanist.

Our most sincere thanks also go to Nikki Bramhill, Director at tfm publishing, for her gentle but firm guiding hand, her tireless work and her enthusiasm and encouragement in bringing this particular project to fruition.

Finally, my personal thanks go to Mrs Sue Cooke, Angela Brooks, Jean Murphy, and Joyce and Ian Keen whose endless efforts over the last 15 years have not only kept The Neuropathy Trust going, but have also been so helpful in ensuring that this new publication becomes available and accessible to all.

Andrew Keen
CEO and Founder, The Neuropathy Trust

Glossary

Acute poliomyelitis: an acute viral disease caused by a poliovirus and marked clinically by fever, sore throat, headache, vomiting, and often stiffness of the neck and back; these may be the only symptoms expressed in the mild form of the illness. In the severe form of the illness, there is neurological involvement, a stiff neck, pleocytosis in spinal fluid, and often infection of bulbar, medullar or spinal muscle motor neurons, with subsequent paralysis and atrophy of corresponding muscles with frequent permanent deformity. Respiratory failure is common requiring prolonged respiratory assistance. Prevention by vaccination is compulsory worldwide.

Allodynia: a condition in which pain arises from a stimulus that would not normally be experienced as painful.

Amyotrophy: muscular wasting or atrophy which can be due to denervation, disuse or cachexia.

Anhydrosis: a deficiency or absence of perspiration.

Areflexia: loss of tendon reflexes.

Ascites: an accumulation of fluid in the peritoneal cavity.

Astereognosia: an inability to identify objects or shapes by palpation.

Ataxia: an inability to coordinate muscle activity during voluntary movement; this most often results from disorders of the cerebellum or from impaired proprioception.

Atony: loss of muscle tone.

Axon: a thin elongated process of a neuron which transmits impulses from the neurone cell body to the axon terminus, which triggers the release of neurotransmitters.

Cachexia: progressive weight loss, anorexia, and persistent erosion of body cell mass.

Campylobacter jejuni: a bacterial species that causes an acute gastroenteritis of sudden onset with constitutional symptoms (malaise, myalgia, arthralgia, and headache) and cramping abdominal pain; potential sources of human infection include poultry and cattle.

Cardiomegaly: increased volume of the heart.

Cardiomyopathy: a disorder of the cardiac muscle.

Castleman disease: a rare disorder characterised by a non-cancerous growth of lymphocytes that may develop at a single site or throughout the body. This disease is similar to lymphoma.

Cauda equina syndrome: a serious neurological condition that manifests with pain, paraesthesia, and weakness involving the L2 to S3 nerve roots making up the cauda equina; there may also be bladder and bowel sphincter dysfunction.

Causalgia: a burning pain, often with trophic skin changes, due to peripheral nerve injury.

Connective tissue disorders: a group of autoimmune disorders in which inflammation affects organs containing connective tissue.

Corti organ: specialised epithelium in the floor of the cochlear duct containing the auditory receptor cells.

Cryoglubulinaemia: a precipitation of immunoglobulins at low temperatures.

Cutis laxa: an increased elasticity of the skin.

Cytomegalovirus (CMV): a member of a group of large species-specific herpes-type viruses with a wide variety of disease effects. It causes serious illness in immunosuppressed people including those at a late stage of infection with human immunodeficiency virus, and in those being treated with immunosuppressive drugs and therapy, especially after organ transplantation. CMV infection produces unique large cells with intranuclear inclusions; the virus can cause a variety of clinical syndromes, collectively known as cytomegalic inclusion disease, although most infections are mild or subclinical.

Dactilitis: an inflammation of an entire digit, as in rheumatoid arthritis.

Delayed-type hypersensitivity reaction: (also called type IV hypersensitivity reaction) a delayed cell-mediated immune response in which CD4+ helper T-lymphocytes recognise a foreign antigen presented by a macrophage. In order to get rid of it they activate natural killer cells, antigen-specific cytotoxic lymphocytes and macrophages, which in turn release cytokines, and form multinucleated cells and granulomas. This kind of reaction occurs in tuberculoid leprosy and in reversal reactions.

Dermatome: an area of skin supplied by sensory neurons that arise from a spinal or a cranial nerve ganglion.

Dysaesthesia: abnormal sensation.

Dysautonomia: a disturbance of autonomic functions.

Dyscrasia: a blood disease or disorder.

Endoneurium: a space located inside the perineurium. It contains nerve fibres, blood vessels, collagen fibres, fibroblasts and endoneurial fluid.

Eosinophilia: an increased number of eosinophilic polymorphonuclear cells.

Epineurium: connective tissue surrounding nerve fascicles.

Episcleritis: an inflammatory condition affecting the episcleral tissue between the conjunctiva (the clear mucous membrane lining the inner eyelids and sclera) and the sclera (the white part of the eye) that occurs in the absence of an infection.

Erythema migrans: an annular rash with central clearing.

Fascicle: nerve fascicle; a bunch of nerve fibres surrounded by a layer of perineurial cells. A nerve root or a nerve trunk is made up of several nerve fascicles.

Fasciculation: spontaneous contraction of a group of muscle fibres.

Ganglion: dorsal root ganglion; an anatomic structure located in dorsal roots, containing the cell body of sensory neurons.

Gastroparesis: delayed emptying of the stomach.

Glucose tolerance test: a metabolic test that measures the ability of the body to metabolise carbohydrates. A patient is administered a standard dose of glucose, and blood and urine samples are measured for glucose levels at periodic intervals following administration. It is used to assist in the diagnosis of diabetes mellitus.

Granuloma: a nodular aggregate of mononuclear cells.

Granulomatosis with polyangiitis: a rare blood vessel disease which can affect the sinuses, lungs and kidneys as well as other organs, usually in association with antineutrophil cytoplasmic antibodies (ANCA) in blood tests.

Helper T-lymphocyte: a sub-group of lymphocytes, a type of white blood cell, that play an important role in the immune system, particularly in the adaptive immune system. They help the activity of other immune cells by releasing T-cell cytokines. They are essential in B-cell antibody class switching, in the activation and growth of cytotoxic T-cells, and in maximising bactericidal activity of phagocytes such as macrophages to form granulomas.

Hemiplegia: paralysis of one side of the body.

Hyperaesthesia: hypersensitivity.

Hyperalgesia: an increased sensitivity to pain, which may be caused by damaged peripheral nerves.

Hyperpathia: a painful sensation in response to a normally innocuous stimulus.

Hyponatremia: a decreased sodium level in the blood.

Hypotonia: decreased muscle tone.

Immunosuppressive drugs: drugs that decrease cellular immunity.

Intravenous immunoglobulin (IVIG): a blood product administered intravenously. It contains the pooled, polyvalent, immunoglobulin G extracted from the plasma of over 1000 blood donors. The effect of IVIGs lasts between 2 weeks and 3 months.

Iridocyclitis: an inflammation of the iris and ciliary body of the eye. The iris is the coloured part of the eye. The ciliary body is the group of muscles and tissues that make fluid in the eye and control movement helping the eye to focus. This condition is also known as uveitis and iritis. It can be caused by the eye's exposure to certain chemicals and various autoimmune disorders.

Ixodes: a genus of hard-bodied ticks.

Lagophthalmos: an inability to close the eyelids completely which exposes the eye to ulceration.

Lepromae: specific lepromatous skin lesions.

Leucopenia: a decreased number of white blood cells.

Leukocytoclasia: destruction of white blood cells.

Lhermitte's phenomenon: electrical sensation that runs down the back and into the limbs elicited by bending the head forward. Originally described in multiple sclerosis.

Light-chain immunoglobulin: the smaller of the two types of polypeptide chains in immunoglobulins, consisting of an antigen-binding portion with a variable amino acid sequence, and a constant region with an amino acid sequence that is relatively unchanging.

Lymphadenitis: inflammation of a lymph node.

Lymphoedema: swelling that develops as a result of an impaired lymphatic system.

Macrophages: white blood cells (activated monocytes) that protect the body against infection and foreign substances by breaking them down into antigenic peptides recognised by circulating T-cells.

Maculae: a spot of skin discoloration.

Meningoradiculitis: meningitis associated with inflammatory lesions of nerve roots in the subarachnoid space.

Mitochondriopathies: sporadic or inherited mutations in nuclear or mitochondrial DNA located genes. Inherited mutations of mitochondrial DNA are associated with a variety of polysystemic manifestations.

Monoclonal gammopathy: an increased production of one type of immunoglobulin by a single clone of cells. The abnormal protein produced is called a paraprotein or an M component and may be composed of whole immunoglobulin molecules or subunits, light chains or heavy chains.

Mononeuritis multiplex: manifestations due to nerve lesions in unrelated portions of the body.

Morton's neuroma: a sharp, burning pain, commonly between the 3rd and 4th metatarsal heads, which is worse with direct pressure and better with rest.

Multinucleated giant cells: large cells with several nuclei resulting from the fusion of activated macrophages in the setting of a delayed-type hypersensitivity reaction.

Multiple sclerosis (MS): an inflammatory demyelinating autoimmune disorder affecting movement, sensation, and bodily functions. It is caused by destruction of the myelin insulation covering nerve fibres in the central nervous system and optic nerves.

Muscle spindles: specialised sensory structures within skeletal muscles, consisting of small muscle fibres which do not contribute to power generation, but participate in muscle control by ensuring a continuous sensory feedback.

Mydriasis: excessive dilatation of the pupil.

Myopathy: a muscle disorder of a genetic or metabolic origin.

Necrosis: tissue destruction.

Neuritis: an inflammatory lesion of a nerve.

Neurofibroma: a benign, non-encapsulated tumour that results from the disorderly proliferation of Schwann cells and that includes portions of nerve fibres.

Neurolymphomatosis: infiltration of the peripheral nervous system by lymphoma and non-tumorous lymphocytes.

Nicotinic receptors: receptors that are stimulated initially and blocked at high doses by the alkaloid, nicotine; they are mainly found on automatic ganglion cells.

Nodes of Ranvier: a short interval in the myelin sheath of a nerve fibre, occurring between each two successive segments of the myelin sheath; at the node, the axon is invested only by short, finger-like cytoplasmic processes of the two neighbouring Schwann cells.

Nucleus pulposus: the central portion of the intervertebral disk that is made up of a gelatinous substance.

Onconeural antibodies: onconeural antibodies are directed against intracellular antigens. They are highly specific markers of a paraneoplastic aetiology in patients with neurological symptoms.

Ophthalmoplegia: paralysis of oculomotor muscles.

Orchitis: an inflammation of the testes.

Osteoarthropathy: a disorder affecting bones and joints.

Osteolysis: dissolution or degeneration of bone tissue.

Osteophytosis: abnormal production of bone as in arthrosis.

Pancoast tumour: tumours that form at the extreme top of either the right or left lung. They tend to invade lower roots of the brachial plexus and the sympathetic chain.

Pandysautonomia: symptoms of widespread and severe sympathetic and parasympathetic failure.

Papilloedema: optic disc swelling that is caused by increased intracranial pressure.

Paraesthesia: painless spontaneous sensation.

Paraneoplastic: changes produced in tissue remote from a tumour or its metastases.

Pericarditis: inflammation of the pericardium, the outer fibrous envelope of the heart.

Perineurium: the connective tissue sheath surrounding each bundle of nerve fibres (fascicle) in a peripheral nerve.

Peripheral neuropathy: signs and symptoms related to lesions of the peripheral nervous system.

Perivascular cuffing: white cells surrounding small blood vessels.

Plasmacytoma: a focal neoplasm containing plasma cells that may develop in the bone marrow, as in multiple myeloma, or outside the bone marrow, as in tumours of the viscera.

Plasmid: a small, circular, double-stranded DNA molecule that is distinct from a cell's chromosomal DNA. Plasmids naturally exist in bacterial cells.

Pleocytosis: the presence of a greater number of cells than normal, as in the cerebrospinal fluid.

Poikilodermia: focal atrophy and telangiectasies of the skin.

Polyarteritis nodosa: a vascular disease that affects the collagen in small- and medium-sized blood vessels inducing necrosis of the arterial wall and lumen occlusion with subsequent ischaemic lesions of affected organs. Polysystemic and constitutional manifestations include multifocal neuropathy, skin lesions, gastrointestinal lesions and kidney lesions. Loss of weight, fever and arthritis are also common. Diagnosis rests on histological demonstration of vasculitis in tissue biopsy specimens. Mortality was high before the use of corticosteroids.

Polycythaemia: an increased number of blood cells.

Proprioception: the ability to sense body position, posture, balance, and motion.

Pseudoathetotic movements: slow involuntary movements of the fingers occurring at rest, associated with a profound loss of proprioception.

Ptosis: drooping of the eyelid.

Retinitis: inflammation of the retina.

Rheumatoid arthritis: a chronic autoimmune inflammatory disease that causes inflammation and deformity of the joints. Pain, swelling, and stiffness in the joints, most often involving the hands, are the main manifestations at onset.

Ribosome: a granule formed of ribonucleoprotein; a site of protein synthesis, under the influence of the nuclear messenger, ribonucleic acid.

Romberg's sign: a loss of balance when the eyes are closed.

Sarcoidosis: a disease associated with granulomas that invariably affects the lungs. In a minority of patients sarcoidosis can become polysystemic and involve other organs including muscles and the central nervous system.

Schmidt-Lanterman incisures: funnel-shaped interruptions in the regular structure of the myelin sheath of nerve fibres.

Schwann cells: cells that form a continuous envelope around each nerve fibre of the peripheral nerves. A Schwann cell enfolds one or more unmyelinated axons. Schwann cells produce a membranous expansion that winds around larger axons to form the myelin sheath.

Schwannoma: a neoplasm originating from Schwann cells. They mostly occur in the skin, but they are also found in nerve trunks and roots.

Spastic paraparesis: weakness of the lower limbs with increased muscle tone and tendon reflexes in relation to lesions of the pyramidal tract in the central nervous system.

Spirochaetes: bacteria that have a distinctive spiral shape.

Syringomyelia: a disorder characterised by damage to the spinal cord, caused by formation of a fluid-filled cavity within the spinal cord, due to trauma, tumours, or congenital defects; the cavity begins in the cervical region and slowly expands. It results in neurological deficits characterised by a dissociated sensory loss (loss of pain and temperature sensation, with preservation of the sense of touch), segmental muscular weakness and atrophy. Thoracic scoliosis is often present.

Systemic lupus erythematosus (SLE): an autoimmune systemic disease that can affect virtually any organ. SLE most often harms the joints, skin, blood vessels, kidney, pericardium and the nervous system. The course of the disease is unpredictable. The disease occurs nine times more often in women than in men.

T2-weighted images: a technique of magnetic resonance imaging that identifies hypersignals in the white matter of the brain in most cases of multiple sclerosis.

T-cells: CD4+ helper T-lymphocytes that are involved in the delayed-type hypersensitivity reaction.

Thrombocytosis: an increased number of thrombocytes in the blood.

Transverse myelitis: an acute attack of spinal cord inflammation resulting in complete paraplegia.

Tropism: attraction.

Type 1 diabetes mellitus: an autoimmune disease characterised by an inability to metabolise carbohydrates, protein, and fat because of absolute insulin deficiency. Type 1 diabetes can occur at any age, but its incidence is more common in children. Uncontrolled type 1 diabetes is characterised by excessive thirst, increased urination, an increased desire to eat, loss of weight, diminished strength, and marked irritability.

Type 2 diabetes: diabetes mellitus, characterised by a late age of onset (30 years or older), insulin resistance, high levels of blood sugar, and little or no need for supplemental insulin.

Uveitis: an inflammation of the middle layer of the eye, called the uvea or uveal tract.

Vascular endothelial growth factor (VEGF): a peptide released from vascular endothelial cells in response to hypoxia, ischaemia, or hypoglycaemia. VEGF promotes proliferation of blood vessels. VEGF is released to maintain the survival of the microvasculature of a tissue.

Vasculitis: inflammatory lesions of blood vessel walls leading to destruction of the vessel wall and occlusion of the lumen.

Voltage-gated channels: ion channels that open and close in response to a change in the electrical potential across the plasma membrane of the cell; voltage-gated sodium channels are important for conducting action potentials along nerve cell processes.

Dedication

This book is dedicated to the memory of
Miss Dawn Louise Ind,
Mrs Olive Briggs
and Miss Dorothea Klyne.

All were neuropathy patients with a
vision of a better future for others.

Chapter 1

Anatomy of the peripheral nervous system

Overview

This chapter is about the different components and functions of the peripheral nervous system which links the central nervous system (brain and spinal cord) to muscles and to sensory receptors for activation of muscle contraction and perception of sensation. The anatomy, motor and sensory territories supplied by plexuses and nerve trunks, and cranial nerves are detailed. The anatomy and function of the sympathetic and parasympathetic nervous systems are also outlined. Microscopic anatomy details the morphology and role of myelinated and unmyelinated nerve fibres.

Introduction

The peripheral nervous system (PNS) has two components: the somatic peripheral nervous system which includes sensory and motor neurons and nerve fibres, and the autonomic nervous system which comprises the sympathetic and parasympathetic systems [1]. The somatic peripheral nervous system controls muscle contraction and perception of sensation, while the autonomic nervous system works automatically without conscious control.

Somatic peripheral nervous system

Each spinal nerve results from the fusion of two roots. The ventral root is formed by the aggregation of spinal motor rootlets (motor neuron axons). The cell body, or perikaryon, of the motor fibre is located in the anterior horn of the spinal cord. The dorsal root contains the dorsal root ganglion, where cell bodies of all sensory neurons of the PNS are found. These two roots unite to form the mixed spinal nerve. There are eight pairs of cervical spinal nerves, twelve pairs of thoracic spinal nerves, five pairs of lumbar spinal nerves, five pairs of sacral spinal nerves and a few pairs of coccygeal nerves.

Cervical plexus

The motor fibre endings of the cervical plexus innervate cervical muscles and the diaphragm. Sympathetic sudomotor and vasomotor fibres pass through this plexus to blood vessels and glands.

Brachial plexus

The brachial plexus is formed by the assembly of C5, C6, C7, C8 and T1 ventral roots. Three trunks (superior, middle and inferior) originate from the brachial plexus. Each of these trunks divides into a ventral and a dorsal branch and three cords are formed (lateral, posterior and medial), which finally lead to the spinal nerves of the upper limbs. The superior brachial plexus is very vulnerable during birth trauma with subsequent deltoid, biceps, brachialis and brachioradialis paralysis. Lower plexus compression by a cervical rib (C8, T1), or infiltration by cells originating from a breast or pulmonary cancer, may cause paralysis of the small hand muscles.

Nerves of the upper limbs

The nerves of the upper limbs are as follows:

- the musculocutaneous nerve (C5, C6) innervates muscles predominantly involved in flexion of the arm;
- the scapular nerve (C5) innervates muscles for elevation and adduction of the scapula;

- the suprascapular nerve (C5-C6) innervates the supraspinatus and infraspinatus muscles for lift and outward rotation of the arm, resulting in abduction of 15° and external rotation of the arm;
- the axillary nerve (C5-C6) innervates the deltoid and teres minor muscles for abduction of the arm to the horizontal and outward rotation of the arm;
- the radial nerve (C6-C8) innervates the triceps, anconeus, brachioradialis, extensor carpi radialis, extensor digitorum and supinator muscles for extension and flexion of the elbow and supination of the forearm; muscles for the extension and flexion of the elbow, supination of the forearm, extension of the wrist and fingers, and abduction of the thumb. Sensory innervation is to the posterior upper arm and forearm, and the posterior thumb and lateral 2½ fingers;
- the median nerve (C5-T1) innervates muscles involved in flexion of the fingers, abduction and opposition of the thumb, and pronation of the forearm. Sensory innnervation is to the palm and fingers 1 to 3 and the lateral half of the fourth finger;
- the ulnar nerve (C8-T1) innervates muscles controlling abduction and adduction of the fingers and wrist flexion; sensory innervation supplies the dorsal and palmar medial faces of the hand, and half of fingers 4 and 5.

Thoracic nerves

The 12 pairs of thoracic nerves give rise to the cutaneous innervation of the thoracic dermatomes. Motor fibres supply innervation of the muscles of the thoracic and abdominal walls.

Lumbosacral plexus

The lumbar plexus is composed of primary branches of the anterior roots L1, L2, L3 and L4. Iliogastric, ilioinguinal and genitofemoral nerves originate from the L1 root and innervate transverse and oblique abdominal muscles. Femoral, obturator and lateral femoral cutaneous nerves are formed from the remaining roots. These nerves are responsible for flexion and adduction of the thigh, leg extension, and sensory innervation of the anterior thigh and leg.

The sacral and coccygeal plexuses are formed from roots coming from L4 to S4. Their main terminal branches are the superior (L4-S1) and inferior gluteal nerves (L5-S2), the posterior femoral cutaneous nerve (S1-S3), the sciatic nerve (L4-S3) and its division into the tibial and common peroneal nerves, and to the pudendal nerve. They result in extension of the thigh, leg and foot, and help to close the bladder and rectal sphincters, and supply sensory innervation of the thigh and perianal region.

Nerves of the lower limbs

The nerves of the lower limbs are as follows:

- the femoral nerve (L2-L4) motor fibres supply the iliopsoas, sartorius and quadriceps femorus muscles resulting in flexion and outward rotation of the lower leg and extension of the lower leg over the thigh; sensory innervation is to the anterior thigh and anterior and medial surfaces of the leg and foot;
- the lateral femoral cutaneous nerve is purely sensory and innervates the anterior and lateral surfaces of the thigh;
- the obturator nerve (L2-L4) controls adduction and rotation of the thigh; cutaneous innervation is on the internal thigh;
- the superior gluteal nerve (L4-S1) controls abduction and inward rotation of the thigh and flexion of the upper leg to the hip;
- the inferior gluteal nerve (L4-S1) motor fibres command extension of the thigh at the hip and outward rotation of the thigh;
- the sciatic nerve (L4-S3) motor fibres supply the biceps femoris, semitendinosus and semimembranosus muscles resulting in flexion of the lower leg, and also muscles dependent upon the tibial and peroneal branches that are terminal branches of the sciatic nerve;
- the posterior femoral cutaneous nerve (S1-S3) supplies sensory innervation of the posterior thigh, lateral perineum and lower buttock;
- the tibial nerve (L4-S2) motor fibres control plantar flexion, inversion of the foot and toe flexion. Sensory innervation is devoted to the lateral calf, foot, heel and small toe;

- the common peroneal nerve (L4-S1) branches to the deep peroneal nerve which gives rise to motor fibres supplying the tibialis anterior, extensor hallucis longus, extensor digitorum longus, extensor digitorum brevis muscles, and to the superficial peroneal nerve, which gives rise to motor fibres supplying the peroneus longus and brevis muscles resulting in foot dorsiflexion and toe extension. Sensory innervation comprises the lateral part of the leg and the dorsal aspect of the foot.

Cranial nerves

The first two pairs of cranial nerves are derived from the cerebrum, while the other ten originate from the brain stem. Cranial nerve I — the olfactory nerve — and cranial nerve II — the optic nerve — do not belong to the PNS. They are actually expansions of the central nervous system (CNS). The other ten cranial nerves enter the PNS after leaving their nuclei in the brainstem.

Oculomotor nerves — cranial nerves III, IV and VI

Cranial nerves IV and VI innervate extraocular muscles only. The third cranial nerve innervates extraocular muscles, the levator palpebrae superioris muscle and pupil constrictor muscle. Complete paralysis of the third cranial nerve induces ptosis, which may totally hide the affected eye, and areactive pupil dilatation (mydriasis).

Cranial nerve IV supplies the superior oblique muscle, allowing the eye to look down and inwards, especially when climbing stairs or reading a book in bed. Cranial nerve VI innervates the lateral rectus muscle, which directs the ipsilateral external gaze.

The trigeminal nerve — cranial nerve V

The trigeminal nerve conveys the sensibility of the face, sinuses, teeth and the anterior part of the oral cavity. It is divided into:

- the ophthalmic branch — pure sensory innervation;

- the maxillary branch — pure sensory innervation; and
- the mandibular branch — sensory and motor innervation of mastication and the tensor tympani muscles.

The sensory part of the ophthalmic division of the cranial nerve V (V1) innervates the cornea and eyeball and forms the afferent limb of the corneal reflex. The maxillary branch innervates the mid-part of the face and the mandibular branch of the lower face.

The facial nerve — cranial nerve VII

The motor fibres of the facial nerve are distributed to the muscles that contribute to facial expression, muscles of the scalp and all facial muscles, and the orbicularis of the eye. Parasympathetic fibres innervate the lacrimal gland and salivary glands. Sensory taste fibres come from the anterior two thirds of the tongue and the soft palate.

The vestibulocochlear nerve — cranial nerve VIII

The utricle, saccule and semicircular canals trigger signals necessary for coordination, balance and movement of the head and neck, which are conveyed through the vestibular component. Expansions of the peripheral spiral ganglion innervate the hair cells along the cochlear duct of the Corti organ. Hearing information from the Corti organ is conveyed to the cochlear nuclei through the cochlear component of the eighth cranial nerve.

The glossopharyngeal nerve — cranial nerve IX

The glossopharyngeal nerve innervates the stylopharyngeus muscle and participates in the innervation of the pharyngeal muscles for swallowing. Sensory fibres convey taste sensitivity of the posterior third of the tongue and posterior part of the soft palate.

The vagus nerve — cranial nerve X

The peripheral motor neurons of the vagus nerve innervate the muscles of the soft palate, pharynx and larynx, allowing speech and swallowing. Preganglionic parasympathetic axons ensure the autonomic parasympathetic innervation of the heart, lung and gastrointestinal tract to the descending colon.

The accessory nerve — cranial nerve XI

The course of the cranial part of the eleventh cranial nerve runs alongside the laryngeal and pharyngeal branches of the vagus nerve and the nerves to the soft palate. The spinal part is formed of spinal motor neurons from the lateral first four or five segments of the cervical spinal cord. The spinal accessory nerve innervates the sternocleidomastoid and the upper two thirds of the trapezius muscles, resulting in the rotation of the head and shoulder elevation.

The hypoglossal nerve — cranial nerve XII

The hypoglossal nerve innervates all the tongue muscles.

Autonomic nervous system

The autonomic nervous system (ANS) consists of efferent fibres that innervate organs such as the heart, smooth muscle, exocrine and endocrine glands, and metabolic tissues, immune cells, etc.; this innervation involves a two-neuron pathway. Afferent activity may travel via the cranial PNS (e.g. vagus nerve) controlled by neurons in the brainstem, or along the somatic PNS (e.g. neurons conveying finger nociception) controlled by neurons of the spinal cord. Thus, sympathetic and parasympathetic preganglionic neurons, which are the first part of the efferent pathway, are activated through interneurons and will synapse with postganglionic neurons that will in turn produce a reflex response (e.g. contraction of vascular smooth muscle in the regulation of blood pressure).

Sympathetic nervous system

The sympathetic nervous system prepares the body for emergency responses. Preganglionic neuron cell bodies of the sympathetic ANS, or thoracolumbar system, are located in the lateral horn of the spinal cord. They leave the spinal cord via ventral roots and terminate either in the lateral ganglionic chain travelling with spinal nerves or in the pre-vertebral ganglionic chain. Preganglionic neurons release acetylcholine (ACh) as the main neurotransmitter in the ganglionic synapse, which activates nicotinic receptors on ganglion cells, allowing a rapid response. Postganglionic sympathetic neurons release the neurotransmitter norepinephrine (adrenergic response) that binds to alpha and beta receptors on targeted tissues. However, postganglionic fibres targeted to the sweat glands release ACh as a neurotransmitter.

Parasympathetic nervous system

This system aims to regulate the repair functions, particularly digestive and elimination functions. Preganglionic neuron cell bodies of the parasympathetic ANS, or craniosacral system, are located in the nuclei of the third, seventh, ninth and tenth cranial nerves and in the intermediate grey matter of the sacral spinal cord S2 to S4, and terminate in visceral or intramural ganglions, near the innervated organ.

Preganglionic neurons release ACh as the main neurotransmitter in the ganglionic synapse, which activates nicotinic receptors on ganglion cells, allowing a rapid response. Postganglionic parasympathetic neurons also release ACh that binds to muscarinic receptors on the targeted tissue.

Microscopic anatomy of peripheral nerves [2, 3]

The nerve trunk is composed of several fascicles, each of which is defined by cylindrical layers of flattened squamous cells forming the perineurium, and embedded in a collagenous matrix, the epineurium which contains blood vessels (Figure 1). Nerve fibres consisting of axons and their associated Schwann cells lie together in these fascicles and are

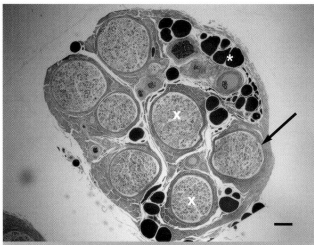

Figure 1. Cross-section of the sural nerve sampled by biopsy to show the multifascicular constitution of a peripheral nerve. The asterisk is positioned in the epineurial nerve compartment which surrounds nerve fascicles. The arrow points to the perineurium, which surrounds and limits nerve fascicles. The crosses are positioned in the endoneurial space, which contains nerve fibres and connective tissue. (Plastic section at 1μm thickness. Thionin staining. Bar: 1mm.)

given mechanical support by endoneurial fibrous collagen and metabolic support from a network of small blood vessels (Figure 2).

The motor neurons and axons

The cell body of motor neurons is located in the anterior horn of the spinal cord and in the motor nuclei of cranial nerves. Motor axons issuing from motor neurons are all myelinated.

Sensory neurons

The cell bodies of sensory neurons are located outside the CNS, in dorsal root ganglia. Two axons are issued from the cell body: one a central branch

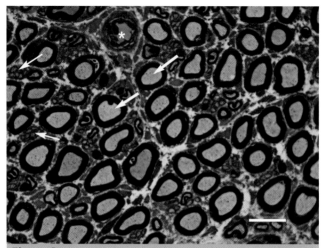

Figure 2. The endoneurium with myelinated and unmyelinated fibres. A one-micron-thick section of a plastic-embedded nerve biopsy specimen showing the myelinated nerve fibres. The unmyelinated fibres cannot be studied by light microscopy. However, they can be seen on this section as pointed out by thin white arrows. The density of myelinated nerve fibres (large arrows) is 7000 to 12,000 per mm² of endoneurial area. The nerve fibre density decreases with age. The density of unmyelinated nerve fibres ranges from 15,000 to 35,000 per mm². An endoneurial blood vessel is marked with an asterisk. (Bar: 10μm.)

which enters the spinal cord with the dorsal root; the other a peripheral branch which travels through the dorsal root, to the plexus and peripheral nerves to reach sensory receptors in the skin, muscles and tendons.

Schwann cells

Schwann cells wrap many layers of tightly packed cell membrane around a single segment of a single axon to form the myelin sheath (Figure 3). Unmyelinated sensory fibres are smaller axons, less then 2μm in diameter. They are surrounded by a single layer of Schwann cell cytoplasmic process. A single Schwann cell wraps several unmyelinated axons.

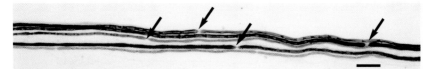

Figure 3. Isolated myelinated fibres. A group of myelinated nerve fibres are isolated by teasing the endoneurial content with fine needles under the microscope. The myelin sheath is grey to black, depending on its thickness, after post-fixation in osmium tetroxide. The nodes of Ranvier are designated by arrows. (Bar: 50µm.)

Nodes of Ranvier

Motor, preganglionic and approximately one third of sensory neurons are myelinated by Schwann cells. Schwann cells wrap many layers of tightly packed cell membrane around a single segment of a single axon, in contrast to CNS myelination where oligodendrocytes wrap multiple layers of tightly packed membrane of a single segment and several adjacent axons. The space between adjacent myelinated segments (or nodes of Ranvier) (Figure 4) contains a high concentration of sodium voltage-gated channels on the axon membrane and allows the reinitiation of the action potential during its spreading on the nerve fibre, from the cell body to the next synapse: this type of conduction is called "saltatory conduction".

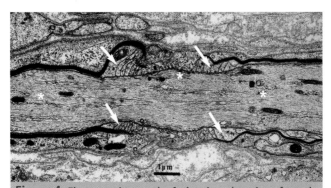

Figure 4. Electron micrograph of a longitunal section of a node of Ranvier. The reflection of the myelin layers on each side of the node are indicated by arrows. The asterisks identify the axon. (Uranyl and lead citrate staining.)

Myelin sheath proteins

The myelin sheath contains several proteins, some the same as found in the Schwann cell plasma membrane and others inserted during compaction of the layers of cell membrane to form the sheath. The myelin protein zero (MPZ, P0) comprises 50-60% of the myelin protein by weight. The small peripheral myelin protein 22 (PMP22) makes up less than 5% of the total protein but is essential for the correct and stable formation of a myelin sheath. Increases in quantity or abnormalities in the structure of this protein underlie a considerable number of inherited peripheral neurological diseases. Found only in the paranode and Schmidt-Lanterman incisures, myelin-associated glycoprotein (MAG) is an important myelin protein, although a very minor component by weight, accounting for only 0.1% of the protein. This is an adhesion protein with five immunoglobulin domains that is only found in non-compacted myelin at the nodes of Ranvier and Schmidt-Lanterman incisures. MAG may be important during the process of myelin formation and may also play a role in the maintenance of the myelin sheath.

Classification of nerve fibres: size, myelination, conduction velocity and function (Figure 5)

This system comprises three groups of fibres (A, B and C):

- group A, the largest fibres with fastest conduction velocities are myelinated somatic afferent and efferent fibres:

  - group A afferent fibres:
  - group I, the largest with diameters of 10-20μm, are sensory afferents from the muscle spindles (Ia) and tendon organs (Ib) with speeds of 50-100m/s;
  - group II (5-15μm, 20-70m/s) include fibres from the secondary endings on intrafusal muscle fibres within the muscle spindle and cutaneous afferent receptors;
  - group III are the smallest myelinated fibres and larger unmyelinated ones with diameters of 1-7μm and speeds of 5-

30m/s. These include nociceptive fibres, sensory afferents from small blood vessel walls and hair follicles;

■ group A efferent fibres:
- α (9-20μm, 50-100m/s) are skeletomotor fibres;
- β (9-15μm, 50-85m/s) are skeletomotor and fusimotor;
- γ (4.5-8.5μm, 20-40m/s) are fusimotor;

● group B are myelinated pre-ganglionic autonomic fibres;
● group C are the smallest, slowest unmyelinated fibres (visceral and somatic afferent and post-ganglionic autonomic efferents).

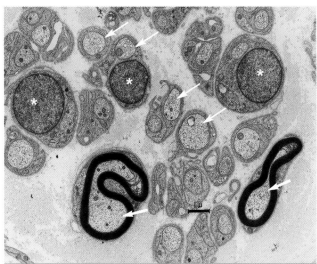

Figure 5. Electron micrograph of a cross-section of a nerve specimen to show the myelinated and unmyelinated fibres, and the Schwann cells. The myelinated fibres are indicated by large arrows and the unmyelinated axons by thin arrows. The asterisks depict the nuclei of Schwann cells.

➲ Key points

- Spinal roots exchange fibres in the cervical and brachial plexuses.
- The cranial nerves provide motor innervation of oculomotor muscles, masticatory muscles, the pharynx, the larynx and tongue muscles.
- Sensory innervation of the face is provided by the trigeminal nerve.
- Nerve trunks destined to the upper limbs are issued from the brachial plexus; those destined to the lower limbs from the lumbosacral plexus.
- The autonomic nervous system is composed of sympathetic and parasympathetic systems.
- The myelinated fibres have larger axons, always surrounded by a myelin sheath made by Schwann cells.
- The unmyelinated fibres are made of smaller axons. One Schwann cell harbours several unmyelinated axons.

References

1. Gardner ED, Bunge RP. Gross anatomy of the peripheral nervous system. In: *Peripheral Neuropathy*, 4th edition. Dyck PJ, Thomas PK, Eds. Elsevier Saunders, 2005: 11-33.
2. *The Peripheral Nerve*. DN Landon, Ed. London: Chapman and Hall, 1976.
3. Staal A, van Gijn J, Spaans F. *Mononeuropathies*. WB Saunders, 1999.

Chapter 2

Basic pathological processes

Overview

This chapter gives a brief summary of the lesions of nerve fibres that occur in different conditions. Axonal degeneration with the Wallerian degeneration component and the dying-back phenomenon are discussed, as is the demyelinating process in some conditions. Also covered is the reparation of lesions of nerve fibres which occurs by sprouting of the axon in axonal neuropathies, by remyelination in demyelinating processes. Finally, general conditions that can affect nerves are outlined, including infection, malignancy and vasculitis.

Introduction

A variety of pathological processes can affect the peripheral nervous system and induce lesions of nerve fibres responsible for signs and symptoms of neuropathy [1, 2]. These processes will be briefly explained in this section and covered in more detail in corresponding chapters.

Pathological processes affecting the nerve fibres

Two main types of degeneration of nerve fibres have been identified — axonal and segmental.

Axonal degeneration

Wallerian degeneration

In this process, the axon is the primary target, inducing secondary degeneration of the myelin sheath, when a myelinated fibre is affected. The injury causing axonal degeneration may act at the level of the cell body of the neuron, in motor neurons located in the anterior horn cell in the spinal cord (in amyotrophic lateral sclerosis for example), or more distally upon the peripheral axon.

When the sensory system is concerned, the cell body of the sensory neuron is located in dorsal root ganglia, where their lesions can induce axonal degeneration of the central and peripheral axonal processes in dorsal roots. Axonal degeneration distal to the lesion is due to separation of the cytoplasm from the nucleus. The first description of the lesions induced by focal trauma to a peripheral nerve is called Wallerian degeneration after Waller (1850) who performed the experiment.

Within a few hours after nerve crush, the distal axon shows signs of degeneration and by 24 hours the myelin sheath starts to split. By 2-3 days the myelin sheath becomes broken into large ovoids within the Schwann cells. The size of the myelin ovoids and balls decrease gradually with time but myelin droplets can still be seen 2-3 months after the nerve lesion.

Simultaneous to myelin degenerative changes, Schwann cells proliferate to prepare the tube that will guide the regenerating axon sprouts which originate from the proximal stump of the damaged axon. Regenerating axon sprouts appear very early, a few days, after nerve crush. They will progress at the rate of fractions of a millimetre to one millimetre per day to reach their target. Regenerating axons are smaller than the original axon and start to myelinate only after reaching the critical size of 1-2μ in diameter. After a few months the regenerated axons form clusters of small myelinated fibres which can be identified on nerve cross-section.

In practice, Wallerian degeneration occurs mainly in traumatic nerve lesions, nerve compression or nerve ischaemia. Another type of axonal degeneration — the dying-back process — is most common in a number of neuropathies.

Axonopathy: dying-back axonal degeneration

Because the peripheral nervous system axons lack ribosomes, the supply of essential structural proteins and enzymes to distal regions (derived from the neuronal perikaryon) must be transported through the axon for great distances. Neurons with long axons are particularly vulnerable to toxic or metabolic disturbances that compromise synthesis or transport of axonal proteins. In toxic neuropathies, diabetic neuropathies and neuropathies due to vitamin deficiencies, sensory and motor deficit predominate in distal lower extremities in relation to degeneration of the terminal parts of the longest axons. This phenomenon called "dying-back" can be due to impairment of the supply of the metabolic requirements from the cell body. The dying-back degeneration is often followed by axonal regeneration by sprouting of the proximal stump (Figures 1-3).

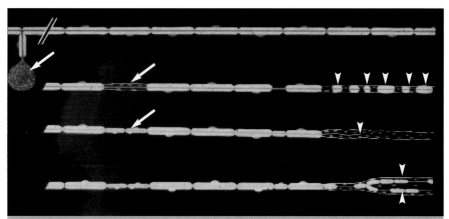

Figure 1. Diagram to illustrate dying-back degeneration. The top row illustrates a normal sensory myelinated fibre with the cell body (arrow). The second row illustrates segmental demyelination (arrow) proximal to distal axonal degeneration with fragmentation of the myelin sheath forming ovoids and balls of myelin containing fragments of axon (arrowheads). The third row shows remyelination of the demyelinated area (arrow) and axonal regeneration by sprouting (arrowhead). The regenerating axon is not yet myelinated. The last row shows a later stage of axonal regeneration with division of the regenerating axon and myelination of axon sprouts (arrowheads).

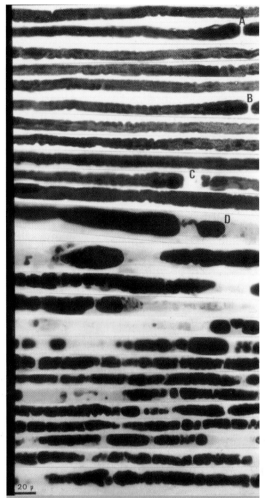

Figure 2. Dying-back degeneration of a nerve fibre in experimental acrylamide intoxication. Consecutive segments of a nerve fibre isolated from the sciatic nerve of a rat intoxicated by acrylamide in drinking water for a month. The proximal end of the isolated segment is at the top left of the panel, the distal end at the bottom right. The myelin sheath is stained black by post-fixation in osmium tetroxide. A and B denotes normal nodes of Ranvier. Distal to node D the myelin sheath shows changes characteristic of Wallerian degeneration.

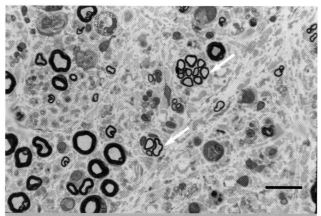

Figure 3. Axonal regeneration. One-micron-thick plastic section of a nerve biopsy specimen from a patient with an axonal neuropathy. Two clusters of regenerating axon sprouts are indicated by arrows. (Bar: 10μm.)

Segmental demyelination

Segmental demyelination is characterised by loss of the myelin sheath between two nodes of Ranvier. Segmental demyelination may result from an immune mechanism as in the Guillain-Barré syndrome or from a toxic mechanism as in diphtheritic neuropathy. The underlying axon is spared and in most instances segmental demyelination is followed by remyelination with replacement of the original internode by several shorter, newly formed internodes. The process of demyelination-remyelination can be completed within a few days or weeks as in the Guillain-Barré syndrome. Demyelinating polyneuropathies are often associated with secondary axonal degeneration which delays or prevents clinical recovery. In diabetic neuropathy, which is the most common neuropathy in the world, segmental demyelination is associated with dying-back axonal degeneration.

Pathological processes affecting nerve blood vessels

Vasculitis, which applies to inflammatory lesions of vessel walls, commonly affects nerve blood vessels, as in polyarteritis nodosa, inducing nerve ischaemia. Blood vessels affected by vasculitis are located in the epineurium. Occlusion of the vessel lumen provokes ischaemia of nerve fibres and massive axonal degeneration. (Please refer to Chapter 6 — Vasculitic neuropathies — for more detail.)

Abnormal deposits in the endoneurium

Endoneurial amyloid deposits cause major and irreversible damage to neighbouring myelinated and unmyelinated nerve fibres responsible for life-threatening familial or light-chain amyloid polyneuropathies. (Please refer to Chapter 10 — Hereditary neuropathies — for more detail.)

Invading malignant cells

Malignant cells can also invade nerve envelopes and provoke degeneration of nerve fibres. Lesions are much more common at the root level than in nerve trunks. (Please refer to Chapter 9 — Neuropathies in patients with monoclonal gammopathy and malignancy — for more detail.)

Infection of the peripheral nervous system

Leprosy is the main infectious neuropathy. Schwann cells are the main target of the infective agent, *Mycobacterium leprae*. Leprosy has been eradicated in developed countries but is still rampant in many areas of Asia, Africa and South America. Neuropathy also occurs in Lyme disease, which is due to *Borrelia burgdorferi*, and in human immunodeficiency virus (HIV) and human T-lymphotropic virus type I (HTLV-1) retroviral infections, but in these conditions the infective agent is not detected in the nerves. (Please refer to Chapter 7 — Infectious neuropathies — for more detail.)

➔ Key points

- Nerve section induces Wallerian degeneration. Dying-back degeneration of axons occurs in length-dependent metabolic or toxic polyneuropathies.
- Segmental demyelination is characterised by loss of the myelin sheath between two nodes of Ranvier.
- Healing of nerve lesions and subsequent clinical recovery occurs by axonal sprouting and remyelination.
- Diabetes and neurotoxic drugs are the main causes of neuropathies associated with dying-back axonal degeneration.
- Segmental demyelination occurs in Guillain-Barré syndrome and chronic inflammatory demyelinating polyneuropathy.
- Lesions of nerve blood vessels, abnormal endoneurial deposits, malignant infiltration and inflammatory lesions can induce massive axonal degeneration of nerve trunks.

References

1.   King R, Ginsberg L. The nerve biopsy: indications, technical aspects, and contribution. *Handb Clin Neurol* 2013; 115: 155-70.
2.   King R. *Atlas of peripheral nerve pathology*. Arnold Publishers Ltd, 1999.

Chapter 3

Clinical manifestations and examination
of patients with peripheral neuropathy

Overview

This chapter breaks down the symptoms of peripheral neuropathy into motor
(mostly weakness), sensory (tingling, numbness and pain) and autonomic
manifestations such as fainting.

The different clinical presentations of neuropathy are discussed and the role of
investigations such as basic blood tests, nerve conduction studies,
electromyography (EMG), and skin, muscle and nerve biopsies are explained.

Symptoms of peripheral neuropathy

As the peripheral nervous system has motor, sensory and autonomic
components, their involvement can lead to various symptoms due to
neuropathy.

Motor manifestations

These include negative manifestations, which are due to loss of
function, or positive manifestations related to hyperactivity of damaged
peripheral motor neurons.

Negative manifestations: motor deficit

Weakness

Damaged peripheral motor neurons lose function, resulting in weakness and muscle atrophy with complete or partial paralysis and amyotrophy. The distribution and tempo of progression of the motor deficit are extremely variable. The onset of the paralysis can be sudden, as in traumatic nerve lesions. In other cases, as in some chronic neuropathies, weakness progresses over years. In such cases muscle atrophy may become obvious long before the onset of weakness. This is often the case in hereditary disorders of the peripheral nervous system. Conversely, in cases with an acute-onset motor deficit, muscle atrophy is observed days to months later after paralysis.

Weakness can affect any nerve territory in the limbs, the trunk or cranial nerves. When predominating in distal lower limbs, the patient complains of tripping on rugs or difficulty in climbing stairs. When predominating in proximal lower limbs the patient will experience difficulty in standing up. When the upper limbs are affected proximally, the patient will notice difficulty in lifting arms up to do their hair. When hand muscles are affected the patient will experience difficulty in turning keys, writing or opening bottles. Minimal weakness of the upper limbs can induce tremor, obvious when the patient outstretches the fingers. Weakness may affect any part of the body including respiratory muscles, the tongue and facial muscles. Depending on the rate of progression and intensity of the deficit, respiratory failure may require respiratory assistance in an intensive care unit.

The power of a muscle or muscle group varies widely and is dependent upon age and gender. Muscle power is usually graded according to the Medical Council Research Scale (Table 1).

Table 1. Medical Council Research Scale.

0:	No contraction
1:	Flicker or trace of contraction
2:	Active movements possible with gravity eliminated
3:	Active movements possible against gravity but not against resistance
4:	Active movements possible against both gravity and resistance
5:	Normal power

Denervation muscle atrophy

Muscle wasting occurs in denervated muscles. It is obvious in most cases but excessive subcutaneous fat may hide the wasting especially in proximal limbs. Wasting of small hand muscles is conspicuous especially when unilateral or asymmetrical (Figure 1). When denervated, the deltoid muscle and/or the quadriceps muscle lose bulk rapidly.

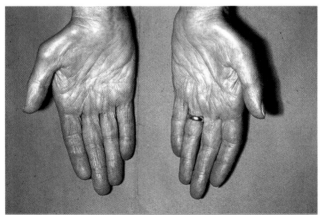

Figure 1. Small hand muscle atrophy in a patient with longstanding compression of the median nerve in the carpal tunnel.

Positive motor manifestations

Positive motor symptoms and signs that accompany peripheral nerve disease, such as fasciculations, myokymia and cramps, occur mainly during active denervation and amyotrophy.

Fibrillation and fasciculation

Fibrillations are spontaneous discharges from a group of single muscle fibres. They result in muscle twitches which are too small to be visible to the naked eye. Fasciculations occur in groups of muscle fibres or in whole motor units. They accompany muscle weakness and atrophy in anterior horn cell disease. Fasciculations, without weakness or muscle wasting, may be a benign phenomenon.

Myokymia and neuromyotonia

Myokymia applies to undulating worm-like localised movements in affected muscles. Myokymia is observed in facial myokymia in multiple sclerosis, and following root lesions or nerve injuries. Neuromyotonia is slow muscle decontraction in a denervated territory.

Segmental myoclonus

Segmental myoclonus consists of rhythmic or semi-rhythmic brisk contractions of muscles innervated by an adjacent spinal or cranial nerve. Myoclonus frequently occurs in post-Bell's palsy or in primary hemifacial spasm, seldom in other sites.

Muscle cramps

Cramps apply to abrupt, usually painful, muscle contraction. They are commonly associated with denervation in motor neuron disease. They are terminated by stretching the affected muscle. Cramps may occur in healthy people without predisposing factors.

Tremor

Postural and action tremors are sometimes observed in the course of a chronic polyneuropathy. It may be disabling. It is typically observed in a territory presenting minimal motor deficit; more often postural tremor affects distal limbs.

Sensory manifestations

Both loss of function and positive sensory manifestations can be disturbing (Figure 2).

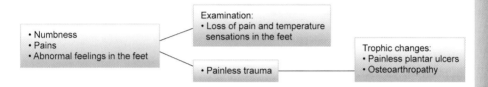

Figure 2. Sensory manifestations.

Loss of function: sensory loss

Assessment during clinical examination
Large myelinated sensory nerve fibres are assessed by testing light touch (cotton), position sense of the large toe and of the fingers. Vibratory sensation is examined with a low frequency tuning fork; temperature sensation is tested by a test tube of warm or cold water. The tendon reflexes are also dependent on large fibre functions.

Pain sensation
Pain can be induced by a range of stimuli. Pinprick is the best way to test pain sensation routinely. The results of sensory tests are consigned to a chart, with one chart for each sensation. Quantitative sensory testing techniques are used to measure sensory thresholds in clinical practice, epidemiologic studies, and therapeutic trials.

Consequences of loss of pain sensation

Distal trophic changes may occur as a non-specific consequence of different congenital or acquired pure or predominantly sensory neuropathies, especially when preserved muscle power makes walking possible.

Trophic ulcers

Perforating ulcers of the foot result from microtrauma on the plantar aspect of the insensitive foot. Blisters can also appear in sensory denervated skin. Trophic ulcers may complicate neuropathy of any origin, leading to sensory loss, with preservation of muscle strength permitting a normal or near normal motor activity. The most common neuropathies responsible for trophic changes include diabetic polyneuropathy, leprous neuropathy, amyloid polyneuropathy, alcoholic polyneuropathy and hereditary sensory neuropathies (Figure 3).

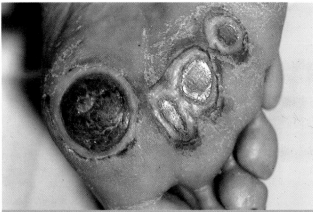

Figure 3. Plantar ulcers at pressure points in a patient with sensory diabetic polyneuropathy.

Osteoarthropathies

Sensory neuropathies may cause osteoarthropathies of the lower limbs. Osteoarthropathy predominates in the feet, up to the ankle, seldom more proximally (Figure 4). In leprosy and in hereditary sensory neuropathies, the fingers can be affected. In syringomyelia, proximal joints of the upper limbs can be affected. Painless fractures, osteolysis and osteophytosis are often associated. Foot deformation and amputation of toes often result from infection, perforating ulcers and osteoarthritis.

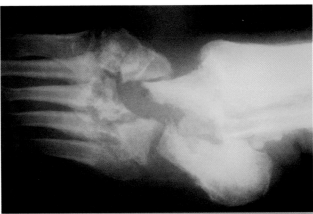

Figure 4. Severe osteoarthropathy in a patient with sensory alcoholic polyneuropathy.

Positive manifestations: spontaneous pains

Pains are the most disturbing symptoms of neuropathy (⊃ see case study overleaf). They are described as burning, tingling, pins and needles, striction (feelings of constriction), walking on rocks, lightning, etc. Pains commonly reveal sensory polyneuropathy. Pain is often worse at night and following activity. It is also made worse by contact — as in causalgia. Often, stimuli which are not normally painful are painful in affected areas; this is called allodynia.

Localisation of symptoms, especially pains, sensory loss and motor deficit are crucial to identify the neuropathic pattern and permit localisation of lesions to a spinal root, as in sciatica; to a nerve trunk, as in median nerve compression in the carpal tunnel. In other cases, the neuropathy is generalised. Each of these patterns of neuropathy requires specific investigation.

Painful peripheral neuropathy

Mark is a 35-year-old right-handed former plumber who had a 5-year history of progressive painful feet that had resulted in him being unable to continue his occupation. His ability to walk had been severely curtailed and he spent his days sitting at home watching TV.

On examination tone and power were normal throughout. Sensory examination revealed a decreased pinprick sensation to three quarters of the way up the forearm of the right arm and to the left elbow. There was decreased pinprick sensation all the way up to the mid-thighs but he had hypersensitivity to pinprick on the soles of his feet. Cold sensation was lost to half way up the forearm bilaterally and half the way up the right shin, and to somewhere above the left knee. Joint position sense was normal in the upper extremities, and reduced in the toes, in that small excursions he did not know which way they were going, but large excursions he did. Vibration sensation was intact. The deep tendon reflexes were all present including ankle jerks, and the plantars were flexor. His gait was slightly wide-based and tentative.

He was thoroughly investigated as to the cause of his neuropathy without an underlying cause being identified. In desperation he was given a trial of steroids on which he improved. Having failed immunosuppressive therapies he was long-term managed on small doses of steroids and intermittent intravenous immunoglobulin with a gradual reduction in his pain over a number of years.

Autonomic dysfunction

Symptoms of autonomic dysfunction are common but are often misinterpreted. Blackouts, faintness and dizziness or visual obscuration on standing are frequent complaints. They reflect the effects of orthostatic hypotension on brain perfusion. They are often associated with some chronic progressive sensory neuropathies. Blood pressure and pulse rate measurement whilst lying, then after one minute in a standing position will detect postural hypotension with a fixed pulse rate.

Neurogenic male impotence is extremely common in diabetic and in amyloid polyneuropathies. It is characterised by the absence of an erection at any time under any circumstances. Neurogenic bladder may present with the complaint of increasing intervals between voiding. Characteristically the patient with a neurogenic bladder has residual urine which is an important risk factor for infection and sepsis. Gastroparesis, diarrhoea and constipation are manifestations of gastrointestinal autonomic neuropathy which may lead to malnutrition and loss of weight.

Distribution of clinical manifestations

Assessment of the distribution of signs and symptoms of neuropathies is crucial to direct further investigations and patient management. The neuropathy can be focal or multifocal, or generalised.

Focal and multifocal neuropathies

Subsequent investigations will depend on the data collected after the first examination (Figure 5). A focal neurological deficit points to lesions of the spinal roots, plexuses or nerve trunks. In this respect the accurate determination of the events that preceded the onset of symptoms is critical since focal root and nerve lesions often result from trauma, compression or wounds. Compression by spinal disc herniation (herniated nucleus pulposus) is a common cause of radicular deficit in the cervical and lumbar regions.

With regard to lesions of nerve trunks, in the upper limbs the radial nerve is commonly affected in the region of the humeral groove. This can occur during unconsciousness from anaesthesia, heavy drinking or during profound sleep. The ulnar nerve is commonly affected by entrapment at the elbow. Entrapment of the median nerve at the wrist level, in the carpal tunnel, is particularly common in older women.

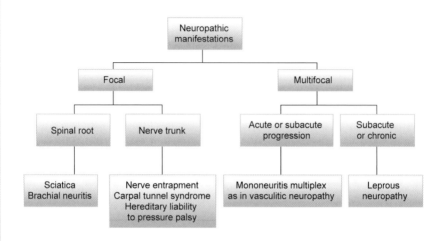

Figure 5. Focal and multifocal neuropathies.

Lesions of the brachial plexus can induce a variety of manifestations. Involvement of the upper portion arising from C5-C7 induces weakness and atrophy of the shoulder and upper arm muscles. Lower brachial plexus involvement (arising from C8, T1) produces distal weakness, atrophy and a sensory deficit in the forearm and hand. The usual causes of upper brachial plexus lesions include trauma, brachial neuritis and damage from radiation. Lower brachial plexus lesions are usually due to malignant infiltration, cervical ribs, brachial neuritis or trauma.

Multifocal deficits are seldom due to multiple root involvement; more often they are due to multiple lesions of the nerve trunk as occurring in leprosy or systemic vasculitis.

Generalised neuropathy

The distribution and pattern of sensory and motor symptoms guide the investigation, differential diagnosis and management of peripheral neuropathies (Figure 6). In generalised polyneuropathies the pattern of sensory loss depends on the type of nerve fibres predominantly involved. When small myelinated and unmyelinated nerve fibres are mainly affected, sensory alteration relating to pain and temperature perception predominates, whilst light touch, position and vibratory senses are preserved. Conversely, when pathology predominantly affects the larger myelinated fibres, proprioception and light touch are affected, often with motor deficits. The distribution of sensory and motor changes is also important.

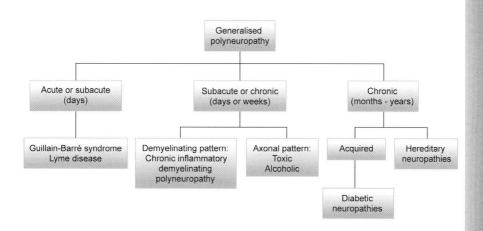

Figure 6. Generalised polyneuropathies.

Length-dependent polyneuropathy

Small fibre neuropathy

In this neuropathic pattern signs and symptoms start and remain more pronounced in the feet, then affect more proximal parts of the lower limbs and eventually the distal upper limbs, which suggests that the longest nerve fibres are affected first. Subsequently, shorter sensory axons are involved, resulting in neuropathic manifestations in more proximal parts of the limbs and eventually the anterior trunk. Pain and temperature discrimination is first impaired in the feet, often leading to painless trauma and plantar ulcers. Loss of temperature discrimination then progresses upward. This is often referred to as a length-dependent pattern and progression of polyneuropathy, which is common in diabetes, but also occurs in alcoholic and amyloid polyneuropathy.

Predominant large fibre involvement

In this setting proprioception is impaired with loss of position and vibratory senses in distal lower limbs. Tendon reflexes are abolished. This pattern of neuropathy is observed in alcoholic polyneuropathy, in paraneoplastic sensory polyneuropathy, or in association with different types of hereditary spinal cerebellar atrophy. In Charcot-Marie-Tooth syndrome (hereditary motor and sensory neuropathy) there is a predominant involvement of larger myelinated fibres that progress following a length-dependent pattern.

Non-length-dependent

In this pattern signs and symptoms affect proximal as well as distal limbs, and even cranial nerves, as in demyelinating polyneuropathy of the Guillain-Barré-Strohl type (Guillain-Barré syndrome). This is an inflammatory, presumably autoimmune demyelinating polyneuropathy affecting the proximal as much as the distal limbs and cranial nerves.

Sensory neuronopathy and sensory ganglioneuropathy are asymmetrical, sensory, painful and ataxic neuropathies, often associated with cancer.

Course of clinical manifestations

The history, neurological pattern and course of the neuropathy are the most important clues to diagnosis. The history of symptoms, background of patients, previous medications, habits concerning alcohol, nutrition, the presence of underlying disorders, and the occurrence of similar symptoms in family members are important. The course of the neuropathy — acute, subacute progressive, relapsing or chronic — is also significant.

Electrophysiological tests

The electrodiagnostic evaluation is an extension of the physical examination. Electrophysiological investigations vary according to the neurological findings on clinical examination. The main purpose of the electrodiagnostic evaluation of peripheral neuromuscular function is to determine the degree, extent and type of pathophysiological changes. Needle electromyography (EMG) and the study of nerve action potentials and conduction contribute to the detection or confirmation of localised nerve lesions. Nerve conduction studies can differentiate between axonal or demyelinating neuropathies, which are important clues to diagnosis.

The main aim of the EMG examination is to determine whether weakness is due to neurogenic involvement or to a muscle disorder as in myopathy. In conventional diagnostic studies the muscle is probed by a concentric needle or by an insulated monopolar needle. The EMG includes recording at rest, weak effort and maximal voluntary contraction. It can be painful for the patient. The findings differ according to the degree of denervation and the temporal profile of the disease. The pattern of denervation in some muscles helps to identify the nerve root, plexus or nerve trunk affected.

Nerve conduction studies are crucial to differentiating between an axonal process with loss of axons — as in Wallerian degeneration — from a loss of myelin in a demyelinating process such as Guillain-Barré syndrome. In routine nerve conduction studies responses are evoked by electrical stimuli and compound responses are recorded from muscles or sensory nerves. The compound muscle action potential (CMAP) is the sum of motor unit action potentials in the muscle. The compound sensory action potential (SNAP) is the sum of action potentials from individual sensory nerve fibres. The amplitudes, shapes and latencies of action potentials change according to the number and function of relevant nerve fibres. SNAPs are about 1000-fold smaller than the CMAPs and usually require averaging (recording multiple events and taking the mean) to increase the signal-to-noise ratio. They are recorded using surface or needle electrodes. Conduction time is assessed by measuring the latency from the stimulus start to the arrival of the response. The amplitude of the SNAP is highly sensitive to axonal loss.

Conventional neurophysiological studies cannot assess the pathophysiology of small myelinated or unmyelinated nerve fibres due to their high threshold to electrical stimulation and the small amplitudes of their action potentials. Degrees of conduction slowing that cannot be explained by fibre loss or axonal atrophy are consistent with demyelination.

Imaging of the PNS

Progress in magnetic resonance imaging (MRI) permits its use in the detection of primary nerve sheath tumours such as schwannomas and neurofibromas. MRI helps to identify the morphological characteristics and spatial extent of spinal roots, and brachial and lumbar plexus lesions to potentially guide the neurosurgical treatment. Imaging can be obtained at entrapment sites, for example, of the median nerve in the carpal tunnel, of the ulnar nerve at the elbow, or in the foot in Morton's neuroma. Ultrasound imaging can also be used to precisely localise lesions of peripheral nerves [1].

Skin biopsy

Skin biopsy is a technique that involves a 3mm punch biopsy of skin taken from standardised sites on the leg. The tissue is immunostained with anti-protein gene product (PGP) 9.5 antibodies. This staining allows for the identification and counting of intra-epidermal nerve fibres (IENF). This technique has been validated as a reliable method for IENF density determination with good intra- and inter-observer reliability in normal controls and patients with a distal symmetrical polyneuropathy [2]. In particular, patients who are suspected of having a predominantly small fibre sensory polyneuropathy may benefit from skin biopsy with IENF analysis since this test can help confirm the diagnosis.

It is common practice to run an immunohistochemical stain for the pan-axonal marker protein gene product 9.5 (PGP 9.5). The sections are then observed and analysed with bright-field microscopy or with indirect immunofluorescence. Most studies report quantification of IENF density displayed in bright-field microscopy. Normative values have been established, particularly from the distal part of the leg, 10cm above the external malleolus. Skin biopsy is of particular value in the diagnosis of small fibre neuropathy when nerve conduction studies are normal. It may also be repeated to study the progressive nature of the disease.

Other diagnostic procedures

Routine blood tests

For most patients, an initial screen blood test should include a complete blood count, erythrocyte sedimentation rate, a comprehensive metabolic panel (blood glucose, renal function, liver function), thyroid tests, serum B12, and serum protein electrophoresis. These blood tests were identified as useful in current evidence-based practice guidelines [3].

Lumbar puncture and cerebrospinal fluid (CSF) examination

Examination of the CSF is an important contribution to diagnosis in many cases. CSF from the lumbar region contains 15-45mg/dL protein and 50-80mg/dL (2.8-4.4mmol/L) glucose (two thirds of blood glucose). Normal CSF contains 0-5 mononuclear cells per mL. The CSF pressure, measured at lumbar puncture (LP), is 100-180mm of H_2O (8-15mm Hg) with the patient lying on their side and 200-300mm with the patient sitting up. The CSF can be diagnostic in meningitis, Guillain-Barré syndrome, Lyme disease and in conditions associated with malignancy when malignant cells can be detected in the CSF [4]. The use of atraumatic needles has been shown to significantly reduce the incidence of post-lumbar puncture headache (3%) when compared to the use of standard spinal needles (approximately 30%). Prophylactic bed rest after lumbar puncture is not mandatory since it has not been shown to be of benefit in some studies.

Indications for nerve biopsy [5]

Progress in neurophysiology and neurogenetics as well as previous neuropathological findings have all improved our knowledge of the pathophysiological characteristics of peripheral nerve disorders. Nerve biopsy is a diagnostic tool which is also an extension of the physical examination and is not just a laboratory test. The indications for nerve biopsy have decreased dramatically during the past decade, making this invasive procedure unnecessary in the vast majority of patients with peripheral neuropathy, but when used judiciously it can be indispensable in diagnosing certain conditions. The yield of nerve biopsy depends on a number of factors, including the selection of patients, expertise of the laboratory, and techniques used, each step being crucial to the usefulness of the procedure.

When performed in unselected patients with peripheral neuropathy, nerve biopsy can be very disappointing because of the lack of specificity of nerve fibre lesions. In addition, patients may complain of discomfort and allodynia (pain from stimuli that normally do not produce pain) for months following the procedure. Before performing a nerve biopsy, the neuropathy must be investigated carefully and characterised by its inheritance, distribution, course, the general context in which it has developed, associated CSF and electrodiagnostic findings, and the availability of DNA testing in the case of hereditary disease.

In hereditary neuropathies, it is now seldom necessary to perform a morphological study of a nerve biopsy specimen.

Acquired, distal, symmetrical, fibre length-dependent polyneuropathies are predominantly sensory and mostly of toxic, especially drug-induced, or metabolic origin. In such cases a biopsy specimen of a distal nerve can indicate the severity and activity of the neuropathy but is unlikely to show any specific lesions, except when amyloidosis is suspected.

In mononeuritis multiplex, a nerve biopsy is required to search for alterations of vasa nervorum, abnormal deposits, or inflammatory infiltrates, many of which are treatable. A whole-thickness nerve biopsy must then be performed under local anaesthesia. Searching for vasculitis is the main indication for a nerve biopsy. The diagnosis of vasculitis should be suspected when a multifocal neuropathy is associated with polysystemic manifestations, but a substantial proportion of patients have isolated neuropathy, sometimes without clinical or biological signs of systemic inflammation. Vasculitis is found in the muscle biopsy specimen in the same proportion of patients in this subgroup as in those with symptomatic multisystemic involvement. Leprosy is still a common cause of neuropathy in subtropical developing countries, but cases of leprous neuropathy are also seen in industrialised countries sporadically. When skin lesions are missing and leprosy suspected, performing a biopsy of an affected nerve is likely to be diagnostic.

Selecting the nerve to biopsy is very important. The nerve should be a sensory nerve in a territory affected by the neuropathic process and easily accessible to neurophysiological studies prior to the biopsy. Performing a biopsy of a nerve in a territory with marked sensory loss decreases the risk of adverse effects and increases the chance of finding significant lesions. Simultaneous muscle sampling increases the chances of finding vasculitis or sarcoid granulomas. Thus, when the neuropathic deficit predominates in distal lower limbs, a biopsy of the sural or superficial peroneal nerve can be performed with simultaneous sampling of an adjacent muscle. After a biopsy of the sural nerve or the superficial peroneal nerve, we prefer to immobilize the leg for 7-10 days to avoid excessive tension over the incision. In patients with proximal involvement of the lower limbs, the intermediate cutaneous nerve of the thigh can be selected and a biopsy of the quadriceps muscle performed during the same procedure. When the upper limbs bear the brunt of the neuropathic process, a biopsy of the superficial radial nerve can be performed at the level of the wrist [6, 7].

⊃ Key points

- Weakness, muscle atrophy, fasciculation, myokymia, cramps and tremor are seen in denervated muscles.

- Sensory loss induces trophic changes, painless osteoarthropathies, and trophic ulcers.

- Different patterns of neuropathy include focal and multifocal neuropathies or generalised length-dependent polyneuropathies.

- Electrophysiological tests are useful to assess axonal loss and nerve conduction slowing in demyelinating processes.

- MRI and ultrasound permit visualisation of nerve and root compression, and tumours.

- Nerve biopsy is indispensable in diagnosing the various conditions.

References

1. Stoll G, Wilder-Smith E, Bendszus M. Imaging of the peripheral nervous system. *Handb Clin Neurol* 2013; 115: 137-53.

2. Gøransson LG, Mellgren SI, Lindal S, Omdal R. The effect of age and gender on epidermal nerve fiber density. *Neurology* 2004; 62: 774-7.

3. England JD, Gronseth GS, Franklin G, *et al*. Practice Parameter: evaluation of distal symmetric polyneuropathy: role of autonomic testing, nerve biopsy, and skin biopsy (an evidence-based review). Report of the American Academy of Neurology, American Association of Neuromuscular and Electrodiagnostic Medicine, and American Academy of Physical Medicine and Rehabilitation. *Neurology* 2009b; 72(2): 177-84.

4. Gorelick PB, Biller J. Lumbar puncture. Technique, indications, and complications. *Postgrad Med* 1986; 79: 257-68.

5. Mellgren SI, Nolano M, Sommer C. The cutaneous nerve biopsy: technical aspects, indications, and contribution. *Handb Clin Neurol* 2013; 115: 171-88.

6. Said G. Indications and value of nerve biopsy. *Muscle Nerve* 1999; 22: 1617-9.

7. King R, Ginsberg L. The nerve biopsy: indication, technical aspects and contribution. *Handb Clin Neurol* 2013; 115: 155-70.

Chapter 4

Guillain-Barré syndrome

Overview

This chapter discusses Guillain-Barré syndrome and its variants. The typical presentation of the syndrome is outlined together with the results of investigations and treatment. The mechanism of demyelination and the role of axonal lesions are described, along with the changes in cerebrospinal fluid and nerve conduction. The need for careful monitoring of autonomic disorders in some patients in intensive care units is underlined. The modalities of treatment with intravenous immunoglobulins and plasma exchange are also described.

Introduction

Guillain-Barré syndrome (GBS) is an acute motor and sensory polyneuropathy with a spontaneously reversible course in most cases. The onset of the paralytic phase is often preceded by a flu-like syndrome. Motor deficit affects all four limbs with frequent involvement of cranial and respiratory muscles, requiring respiratory assistance. Increased cerebrospinal fluid (CSF) protein content and reversibility of neurological deficit characterise the syndrome. Several variants have been added to the classical description of the syndrome, which in most cases have a favourable outcome. Disabling sequelae remain relatively common, however.

Historical background

GBS was originally described, almost one hundred years ago, by Guillain, Barré and Strohl as a peculiar flaccid paralysis in two soldiers who had developed acute paralysis with areflexia, from which they recovered spontaneously [1]. The neurological deficit is typically associated with increased protein concentration in the CSF with a normal cell count.

GBS is a post-infectious, inflammatory and demyelinating peripheral neuropathy (also called acute inflammatory demyelinating polyneuropathy), but forms with predominant axonal damage have subsequently been identified. Such axonal forms of GBS, called acute motor axonal neuropathy (AMAN) or acute motor and sensory axonal neuropathy (AMSAN), are more common in some countries such as China after infection by *Campylobacter jejuni* [2].

The latest overall estimation for the frequency of this disorder is 1.1 to 1.8 per 100,000 persons per year. GBS is now, in the post-polio era in developed countries, the most frequent cause of acute paralysis, potentially life-threatening, and occasionally lethal [3].

Pathophysiology

Following non-specific infection, vaccination or a surgical procedure, patients may develop a GBS due to acute demyelination of spinal roots and nerve trunks, without significant axonal involvement in most cases [4]. This demyelination results from an autoimmune process mediated by macrophages activated by helper T-lymphocytes directed against components of the myelin sheath. Acute demyelination can also result from antibodies induced by the infection, cross-reacting with antigens of the myelin sheath. Both mechanisms lead to acute demyelination with its consequence of impaired function of axons. Acute demyelination of groups of nerve fibres can induce conduction block, and paralysis of corresponding territories. Demyelination and conduction block are the physiological bases of neurological deficits in GBS. Recovery from GBS paralysis can be relatively rapid, taking a few days to a few weeks, although in some cases it may extend over several months. The demyelinating process, however, is characteristically self-limiting in GBS, and remyelination is a rapid process with subsequent recovery of normal conduction and suppression of conduction block and paralysis. Since axonal continuity and function are preserved recovery can be complete. In some cases, however, there is bystander axonal damage which may lead to a more protracted course and sequelae.

In some cases axonal lesions predominate, as in the so-called acute motor axonal neuropathy (AMAN) or acute motor and sensory neuropathy (AMSAN), which have the same course as GBS but with a poorer outcome. Since demyelination is not a feature of this form of neuropathy, electrophysiological investigations will show only axonal damage without nerve conduction slowing or conduction block. Intermediate forms are common, however. The axonal forms are more common in some countries, especially in China, following gastrointestinal infection with *Campylobacter jejuni*. This bacterial infection is common but actually induces GBS in less than 0.1% of infected people. Host factors are likely to influence the susceptibility to GBS.

Clinical aspects

Since the virtual disappearance of acute poliomyelitis, GBS is the most common acute areflexic quadriparesis. Typically, about two thirds of patients give a history of recent acute infection, a flu-like syndrome or a mild respiratory syndrome; occasionally the onset of GBS follows seroconversion to HIV infection. Post-surgical GBS, which accounts for approximately 5% of GBS patients, occurs 2-3 weeks after the surgical procedure.

Distal paraesthesias, numbness and pain usually herald the start of the illness. Weakness can start equally in the upper and lower limbs, or affect the lower limbs or the upper limbs first (⮕ see case study overleaf). Inaugural sensory symptoms and paraesthesias are associated with pain in 50% of patients, but as many as 90% of patients eventually complain of pain [5]. Weakness may affect the neck and pharyngeal muscles. Bilateral symmetrical facial weakness — facial diplegia — occurs in more than 50% of cases. Partial or complete paralysis of oculomotor muscles

Guillain-Barré syndrome

Ian is a 27-year-old painter and decorator who was admitted to the neurology service at 22:00 having gone up to casualty with severe pain in his legs which had developed over the course of the day. He had become unsteady on his legs. He was admitted overnight and the junior staff could not decide what was wrong with him, but having identified weak legs with normal reflexes had organised an MRI scan of the spine for the following morning. On the morning ward-round the consultant found no abnormality in the arms, but his legs were weak generally in the 4/5 range. There was a loss of vibration sensation in the toes and a minor impairment of proprioception. His ankle jerks were absent with flexor plantar responses. He was in significant pain. A diagnosis of GBS was made and he was started on intravenous immunoglobulin (IVIG) at a dose of 0.4g/kg daily for 5 days. The subsequent MRI of the complete spine was normal. His CSF was normal apart from a mildly elevated protein level, and the peripheral electrophysiology performed within 2 days of presentation was normal.

The pain settled over the next 4 days and his walking gradually improved. He was discharged from hospital within a week of arrival and was able to return to work 6 weeks after his initial presentation, though he struggled with fatigue.

(ophthalmoplegia) occurs in 3-5% of patients. The weakness reaches a maximum state at 2-4 weeks after symptom onset, with progressive recovery over weeks to months.

Patients with GBS initially exhibit few objective signs besides weakness. Sensory signs are usually limited to glove and stocking hypoaesthesia to light touch. Position sense and a decrease of vibratory sensation are often impaired after a few days. Examination shows flaccid paraparesis or paraplegia, with a loss of tendon reflexes and mild sensory changes in most cases. Dysautonomia occurs in 15% of patients, including cardiac arrhythmia, hypertension or hypotension, ileus and urinary retention [6]. In some individuals, respiratory failure may occur early, while others may have no respiratory involvement, so the extent and distribution of the symptoms vary greatly among individuals with GBS.

In the classical form of GBS, lesions of roots and nerves are characteristically demyelinating while the underlying axons are relatively spared. In the axonal variant, the axons are predominantly involved. The course seems more rapid and severe in the axonal form of GBS, with more frequent and severe respiratory and cranial nerve involvement. Dysautonomia is less common in the axonal pattern. Preceding *Campylobacter jejuni* infection seems more common in the axonal variants than in classical GBS. The AMAN form is a pure motor syndrome, while AMSAN is characterised by both motor and sensory deficits. The latter is thought to be the more advanced or severe form of axonal subtypes.

The ophthalmoplegia, ataxia and areflexia syndrome or Miller-Fisher syndrome

Miller-Fisher syndrome (MFS) is a cranial nerve variant of GBS, characterised by the presence of ophthalmoplegia, ataxia and areflexia [7]. There is no motor involvement but considerable impairment of balance due to impaired proprioception. Ophthalmoplegia is characterised by paralysis of ocular muscles. The loss of tendon reflexes is related to the involvement of large sensory myelinated fibres. MFS is generally regarded as a self-limiting disorder; however, some patients may require respiratory assistance. Complete recovery is the rule in MFS.

Diagnosis

The diagnosis of GBS and variants rests on the clinical pattern and electromyography (EMG) and CSF. Characteristically, the neurological deficit is not 'length-dependent'; that means that it does not affect the longest fibres and distal limbs first. Also it is predominantly motor with little or no sensory loss. A decrease in light touch sensation, alteration of proprioception and loss of tendon reflexes all point to the involvement of larger myelinated fibres.

CSF examination after lumbar puncture is a key contribution to diagnosis. CSF protein concentration is raised in 80% of patients, sometimes several times the upper limit of normal values, while the mononuclear cell count is usually normal as described by Guillain *et al* [1]. The CSF protein level may remain normal in a small proportion of patients and may be normal early on in the illness.

In the early stages, particularly before areflexia is present, it may be necessary to undertake magnetic resonance imaging (MRI) of the spinal cord to exclude a transverse myelitis or cord compression which can mimic the presentation of GBS.

The classical findings of nerve conduction studies include the presence of a partial motor conduction block, an abnormal temporal dispersion of motor responses, prolonged distal motor and F-wave latencies, and reductions in maximum motor conduction velocity. Nerve conduction studies may be normal initially, and sometimes remain normal subsequently, because the territories explored by conduction studies are not affected by the disease. In territories with motor deficit, however, needle EMG will detect non-specific denervation. Repeated electrophysiological tests and CSF examination during the course of the paralytic or recovery phase of the disease are not necessary, except for research purposes.

Pathology

The pathology of GBS has been described in the seminal findings by Asbury *et al* [8]. Lesions predominate on spinal roots. The associated inflammatory infiltrates consist of lymphocytes and macrophages with a resulting demyelination. Macrophages infiltrate the myelin sheath and strip myelin layers to demyelinate the underlying axon. Lesions often predominate on anterior roots. Most axons remain intact in the demyelinated area. Due to the intensity of the inflammatory process, however, or to specific antibodies to axonal components, the axon can be damaged with subsequent axonal degeneration, which precludes rapid remyelination and alleviation of the conduction block induced by acute demyelination (Figures 1-4) [9].

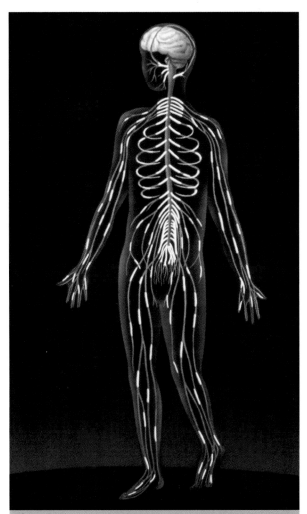

Figure 1. This schema shows the distribution of demyelinating lesions in GBS. Demyelination predominates in proximal parts of the peripheral nervous system. They are often patchy, especially in nerve trunks.

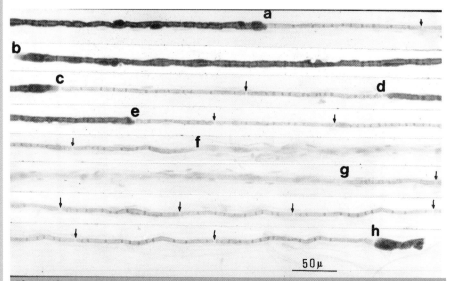

Figure 2. Consecutive segments of a nerve fibre isolated from a nerve biopsy specimen of a patient with Guillain-Barré syndrome to show segmental demyelination. The myelin sheath is stained in black by post-fixation in osmium tetroxide. The myelin sheath has normal thickness from top left to the node of Ranvier a and then from b to c and d to e. Between f and g the fibre is completely demyelinated while the other segments are thinly remyelinated (arrows).

In the axonal variants of GBS, the lesions predominate on axons and occasionally on neurons (Figure 4) which accounts for clinical and electrophysiological features and badly impairs recovery.

Prognosis and evolution

In relation to the self-limiting underlying pathological process, namely acute segmental demyelination, the outcome of GBS is spontaneously good in most cases, within a few weeks, as emphasised in the original description [1]. Remyelination of affected portions of roots and nerves is a rapid phenomenon, which quickly alleviates conduction block permitting a return of normal function and clinical recovery within a few weeks in most cases. After the initial phase of progressive paralysis, the patient enters a

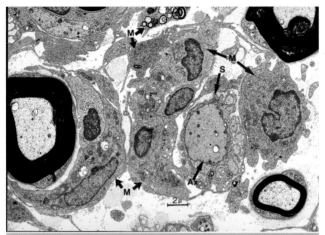

Figure 3. Electron micrograph of a nerve biopsy specimen from a patient with GBS to show a demyelinated axon (Ax) surrounded by macrophages (M) which are removing myelin debris from the demyelinated axon. S = Schwann cell. (Uranyl acetate and lead citrate staining.)

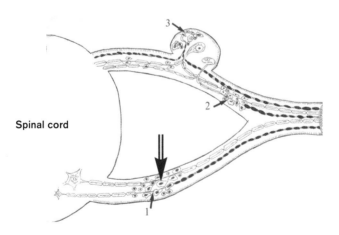

Figure 4. This schema illustrates the sites of axonal involvement in GBS. The large arrow points to a demyelinated fibre in the ventral (anterior) root, which contains motor fibres. Arrows 1 and 2 point to axonal lesions of nerve fibres in the anterior and posterior roots, respectively. Arrow 3 points to a lesion of the cell body of sensory neurons in a dorsal root ganglion.

plateau phase of varying duration, which ranges from days to several weeks or months. This phase is followed by a recovery phase of varying duration.

GBS is generally regarded as a monophasic illness but about 10% of patients show a re-deterioration or relapse. In Europe, about one third of patients with GBS remain able to walk (mildly affected patients) during the plateau phase. In patients with GBS who are admitted to hospital and are unable to walk (severely affected patients), about 25% need artificial ventilation, mainly because of respiratory muscle weakness. Twenty percent of patients requiring mechanical ventilation die, and the recovery of most survivors is a prolonged process. Otherwise, in spite of the effect of intravenous immunoglobulin or plasma exchange treatment (see below), about 20% of severely affected patients remain unable to walk after 6 months [10]. Moreover, many patients remain disabled or have severe fatigue. It is noteworthy that GBS has a significant negative impact on social life and daily activities, even 3-6 years after onset. Of the totality of patients with GBS, 3-10% will die, and in some of these patients the cause is likely to be (sudden) autonomic failure with cardiovascular instability. Age greater than 50 and disability due to prominent axonal lesions are the main indicators for a poor prognosis with regard to walking at 6 months.

Treatment

Patients with GBS need integrated multidisciplinary care to prevent and manage potentially fatal complications. Patients need careful monitoring of respiratory function, including vital capacity, respiration frequency, blood gases, and possible autonomic dysfunction, such as heart rate, arrhythmia, and blood pressure. Infections and deep vein thrombosis need to be prevented. The recognition of autonomic dysfunction (ileus, pupillary light reflex) is required alongside the management of pain, physiotherapy, rehabilitation and psychological support for severely affected patients.

The presumed autoimmune mechanism of GBS has led to immunomodulating treatments, which seem to shorten recovery time, without preventing residual deficits in all patients [11]. In mildly affected patients there have not been any placebo controlled trials, to date, assessing the effect of plasma exchange (PE) or intravenous immunoglobulin (IVIG) in these patients with GBS.

The latest review on the use of PE in GBS (2008) stated:

- in mild Guillain-Barré syndrome, two sessions of plasma exchange are significantly superior to one;
- in moderate GBS, four sessions are significantly superior to two;
- in severe GBS, six sessions of plasma exchange are not significantly better than four;
- plasma exchange is more beneficial when started within 7 days of disease onset rather than later, but was still beneficial in patients treated up to 30 days after disease onset [12].

Intravenous immunoglobulin in a regimen of 0.4g/kg body weight daily for 5 consecutive days has replaced PE as the preferred treatment in many centres, mainly because of its greater convenience and availability. The latest Cochrane review stated significant benefits of IVIG in [12]:

- improvement in disability grade, 4 weeks after treatment;
- shortening the time to recovery of walking unaided; and
- shortening the time to discontinuation of artificial ventilation.

Guillain Barré syndrome is a self-limiting inflammatory, autoimmune, demyelinating polyneuropathy. GBS has a good overall prognosis, with spontaneous complete recovery in most cases, within a few weeks or months. Fatal outcome is very rare but sequelae that include motor deficit, sensory loss or pain remain relatively common, in spite of modern immunotherapy.

➔ Key points

- Pain and weakness occur at the onset of Guillain-Barré syndrome.
- Clinical manifestations of Guillain-Barré syndrome are best explained by the interruption of axonal function by conduction blocks.
- The Miller-Fisher syndrome is associated with ophthalmoplegia, ataxia and areflexia. It has a favourable outcome.
- Axonal involvement delays recovery from GBS.
- Patient management in the intensive care unit should include physiotherapy and psychological support.
- Plasma exchange and intravenous immunoglobulin treatment must be used early in the course of GBS.

References

1. Guillain G, Barré J, Strohl A. Sur un syndrome de radiculonévrite avec hyperalbuminose du liquide céphalorachidien sans réaction cellulaire. Remarques sur les caractères cliniques et graphiques des réflexes tendineux. *Bull Soc Med Hop Paris* 1916; 28: 1462-70.

2. McKhann GM, Cornblath DR, Griffin JW, *et al*. Acute motor axonal neuropathy: a frequent cause of acute flaccid paralysis in China. *Ann Neurol* 1993; 33: 333-42.

3. McGrogan A, Madle GC, Seaman HE, *et al*. The epidemiology of Guillain-Barré syndrome worldwide. A systematic literature review. *Neuroepidemiology* 2009; 32: 150-63.

4. Fujimura H. The Guillain-Barré syndrome. *Handb Clin Neurol* 2013; 115: 383-402.

5. Moulin DE, Hagen N, Feasby TE, *et al*. Pain in Guillain-Barré syndrome. *Neurology* 1997; 48: 328-31.

6. Kuwabara S. Guillain-Barré syndrome: epidemiology, pathophysiology and management. *Drugs* 2004; 64: 597-610.

7. Fisher M. An unusual variant of acute idiopathic polyneuritis (syndrome of ophthalmoplegia, ataxia and areflexia). *N Engl J Med* 1956; 255: 57-65.

8.   Asbury AK, Arnason BG, Adams RD. The inflammatory lesion in idiopathic polyneuritis.
      Its role in pathogenesis. *Medicine (Baltimore)* 1969; 48: 173-215.

9.   Prineas JW. Pathology of the Guillain-Barré syndrome. *Ann Neurol* 1981; 9 (Suppl): 6-
      19.

10.   Hughes RA, Swan AV, Raphael JC, *et al.* Immunotherapy for Guillain-Barré syndrome:
      a systematic review. *Brain* 2007; 130: 2245-57.

11.   Lehmann HC, Hartung HP. Plasma exchange and intravenous immunoglobulins:
      mechanism of action in immune-mediated neuropathies. *J Neuroimmunol* 2010; 231:
      61-9.

12.   Raphaël JC, Chevret S, Hughes RA, Annane D. Plasma exchange for Guillain-Barré
      syndrome. *Cochrane Database Syst Rev* 2012; 7: CD001798.

Chapter 5

Chronic inflammatory demyelinating polyneuropathy

Overview

Chronic inflammatory demylinating polyneuropathy (CIDP) has some similarities to Guillain-Barré syndrome (GBS) but progresses over a longer period (more than a month) and requires different treatment. The different patterns of CIDP are outlined, including the relapsing and progressive forms, as well as a purely sensory neuropathy at the onset. Other subjects covered are CIDP in diabetic patients, the association of CIDP with monoclonal gammopathy of unknown significance, and the polyneuropathy, organomegaly, endocrinopathy, monoclonal gammopathy and skin changes (POEMS) syndrome with plasmacytoma. Treatment with corticosteroids, intravenous immunoglobulins, plasma exchange and immunosuppressive drugs are also discussed.

Introduction

Chronic inflammatory demyelinating polyneuropathy (CIDP) is an acquired peripheral neuropathy, presumably of immunological origin. Its clinical presentation and course are extremely variable. Diagnosis should not be missed because it is one of the few peripheral neuropathies that responds well to treatment.

CIDP is characterised morphologically by longstanding multifocal demyelination that predominantly affects spinal roots, major plexuses and proximal nerve trunks.

Epidemiology

The crude prevalence of CIDP is approximately 1 to 2 per 100,000 population. The mean age of onset is around 50 years, but it may occur at any age. CIDP is the second most common cause of disabling neuropathy in the elderly. The stringent electrophysiological criteria defined by the American Academy of Neurology Ad Hoc Subcommittee research criteria for the diagnosis of CIDP underestimates the real incidence of CIDP [1].

Clinical manifestations

The diagnosis of CIDP may be made when a patient presents with a non-fibre-length-dependent demyelinating polyneuropathy that progresses over more than a month, or evolves chronically over many months. The subsequent course can be progressive, or relapsing and remitting, often with a secondary progressive course. The underlying demyelinating process needs to be demonstrated by electrophysiological studies or occasionally by nerve biopsy [2].

Precipitating factors

There is no identified genetically determined susceptibility to CIDP. A history of an illness, mostly non-specific upper respiratory or gastrointestinal tract infection, or vaccination in the preceding 6 months was reported in one third of cases. Different patterns of CIDP, relapsing or progressive, have been observed at all stages of HIV infection.

Neurological manifestations at onset

The manifestations at onset are extremely variable. In the generalised pattern the presentation includes numbness of the upper and lower extremities, spontaneous pain and weakness that progress gradually over several weeks (⟳ see case study overleaf). In some cases a progressive sensory ataxia is the presenting manifestation, while in others a predominantly or purely motor deficit is observed at onset. In most cases

Chronic inflammatory demyelinating polyneuropathy

Gillian is a 52-year-old diabetic nurse who developed lumbar back pain, which became severe. Imaging revealed an old crush fracture and she was admitted to an orthopaedic ward. After a couple of weeks she was transferred to a rehabilitation facility. She developed a band-like sensation round her lower thoracic region and by the time she was discharged home from the rehabilitation facility after 3 weeks, she was bent over and unable to walk without the assistance of a stick. She was seen by a senior colleague, 2 months after the onset of her symptoms, who found a normal neurological examination apart from a relative diminution in the knee and ankle deep tendon reflexes. However, he was significantly worried about her deterioration and arranged for her admission to the neurology service a couple of days later. She was re-examined by the admitting attending neurologist who found hip flexion weakness in the 4/5 range, normal power at the knees, but weakness of dorsiflexion of the feet in the 4+/5 range and her deep tendon reflexes were absent at her knees and ankles. The plantar responses were flexor. A clinical diagnosis of chronic inflammatory demyelinating polyneuropathy was made, which was confirmed by her cerebrospinal fluid (CSF) showing an elevated protein of 0.95g/L and the peripheral electrophysiology confirming demyelination. She was started on 0.4g intravenous immunoglobulin per kg per day for 5 days. Within a week she had significantly improved and was able to ambulate. Further treatment will be initiated, such as steroids and azathioprine, if she fails to continue to improve or deteriorates.

the deficit is roughly symmetrical, both proximal and distal. In other cases focal or multifocal involvement produces a multifocal demyelinating neuropathy with or without conduction block on electrophysiological testing. At onset, the incidence of motor deficit varies from 78-94% of the cases as illustrated in three large studies [3-5]. In McCombe's study a gradual onset of symptoms occurred in 84% of patients, while in 16% the onset was acute, with the plateau of disability being reached within 4 weeks. In many cases, the diagnosis of CIDP is made retrospectively because of the subsequent relapsing or progressive course, or secondary involvement of other nerve territories.

Neurological manifestations at steady state

The clinical manifestations at the chronic phase, steady state, or at referral, reflect the extreme symptomatic variety of CIDP. On average motor deficit occurs in 83-94% of patients and sensory deficit in 72-89%. Facial palsy is observed in 4-15% and loss of tendon reflexes in 86-94% of patients. Dysautonomia is not a feature of CIDP.

Increased CSF protein content

Increased CSF protein content is a major feature in CIDP. Some authors have made it mandatory for diagnosis that there be a CSF protein content of more than 0.45g/L, with less than 10 cells per ml. In our studies, the CSF protein content was normal in 14% of patients and cellularity was normal in all of them. When the CSF is normal, it is mandatory to support the diagnosis with unequivocal demyelinative features on electrophysiological tests or pathological data.

Clinical variants of CIDP

Clinical diversity in the presentation and course are the most remarkable features of CIDP.

Focal and multifocal neuropathy and CIDP

Chronic inflammatory demyelinating polyneuropathy presents in rare instances with focal or multifocal upper limb involvement. Symptoms can begin in one arm or hand, or in both arms or hands with paraesthesias, weakness, and pain [6].

Findings can be initially restricted to the one nerve distribution or involve multiple nerves. Aside from the focal onset, there is no difference between focal and generalised CIDP.

Chronic sensory demyelinating polyneuropathy

Some patients present with isolated sensory manifestations, including ataxia, pain, and paraesthesias of the lower extremities, which represent a subset of CIDP. Two groups of patients can be identified in those presenting with isolated sensory manifestations. In the first group, sensory manifestations are followed after a variable period of time by motor deficit. In the second group the signs and symptoms remain purely sensory for years or decades. In our study of 28 patients with isolated sensory manifestations at onset, five developed motor deficit on average 4.5 years after the onset [7]. In the remaining patients the neuropathy remained purely sensory after a mean follow-up of 7.2 years. Large fibre function was impaired in all patients; pain and a loss of temperature sensation was found in 90% of cases. The mean CSF protein level was 0.77g/L, but the CSF was normal in 12 (44%) patients. At least one motor conduction parameter, including motor conduction velocity (MCV) and F-wave distal latency, was in the demyelinating range in 96% of patients. Conduction block and temporal dispersion were found in 30% of patients. The course was progressive from the onset in 22 patients (81.5%), secondary progressive in one, and relapsing in four (15%). Disability, which was mainly due to ataxia and loss of tactile discrimination, was present at referral in 26% of patients. Improvement was noted in 8/15 (53%) patients treated with oral prednisone and in 4/14 (29%) patients treated with intravenous immunoglobulins (IVIGs).

Pure motor pattern

Pure motor patterns are observed in the same proportion of patients as pure sensory forms. In some cases ventral roots bear the brunt of demyelination, as is often the case in GBS.

CIDP in childhood

CIDP is rarer in children than in adults but the clinical aspects, course and response to treatment are similar to that in adult-onset CIDP. In a study comparing 12 children with idiopathic CIDP to 62 adults with idiopathic CIDP, Simmons and coworkers found that children often had more rapidly fluctuating courses than adults; a relapsing course was significantly more common in children than in adults [8]. The recovery of children from each episode of deterioration was usually excellent and better, on average, than in adults.

CIDP in diabetic patients

Patients with diabetes occasionally develop clinical and electrodiagnostic features suggestive of CIDP. This diagnosis must be suspected when a predominantly motor and ataxic polyneuropathy occurs in a diabetic patient. In one study of diabetic patients with CIDP, the nerve conduction studies showed more severe axonal loss and the degree of improvement following treatment was less favourable [9].

Postural and action tremor in CIDP

Postural and action tremors can become a very disabling symptom in patients with CIDP. Such tremors occur in patients with minimal motor weakness regardless of the intensity of sensory manifestations. Increased physiological tremors are related to weakness with a possible role of decreased input from afferent large myelinated fibres.

Central nervous system (CNS) involvement in CIDP or CIDP and multiple sclerosis (MS)

CIDP was associated with symptomatic lesions of the CNS in 5% of cases in our series [3]. Imaging characteristics of MS were found in the three patients who underwent magnetic resonance imaging (MRI). All patients with CNS involvement were severely handicapped.

Clinical course and prognosis

The long-term outcome of CIDP is unpredictable in the early stages of the disease. A variable proportion of cases follow a relapsing or chronic progressive course, with many patients starting with a relapsing course followed by a secondary progressive course. In that respect CIDP can be considered a peripheral analogue of MS. In addition, just as in MS, loss of axons is a major negative prognostic factor identified in CIDP.

Bouchard *et al* reviewed the follow-up data of 83 patients collected 6 years on average after the first manifestations of neuropathy [3]. The outcome was good in 56% of patients. Nine patients died as a result of progression of the neurological deficit to quadriplegia, and respiratory and swallowing difficulty. The mean age of patients who died was 67 years. Relapsing forms carried a better prognosis than progressive forms, in keeping with a better response of patients with acutely relapsing CIDP to IVIG treatment. A relapsing and remitting course predominated in the juvenile group. Functional recovery was common in all age groups, but was the least apparent in the elderly group.

Electrophysiological data

The main purpose of electrophysiological studies in patients suspected of CIDP is to establish the presence of focal, multifocal, or diffuse demyelination, and to ascertain the anatomical extent and distribution of abnormalities. In practice, the diagnosis of CIDP rests mainly on demonstration of an asymmetrical demyelinating process, and patients with acquired demyelinating neuropathy often have a differential slowing of conduction velocity when proximal and distal latencies of equivalent segments of two nerves in the same limb are compared.

Criteria for CIDP include:

- motor conduction velocity of less than 75% of the lower limit of normal values;
- distal motor latencies greater than 140% of normal values;
- conduction block and/or temporal dispersion of the compound muscle action potential;
- increased F-wave latency to greater than 120% of normal.

Electrophysiological tests, although crucial for the diagnosis of demyelinating polyneuropathies, do not yield clear-cut results in many cases, due to the mixture of axonal loss with demyelinative features in patients with primarily demyelinating neuropathies. Nerve biopsy should be considered when a clinical suspicion of an inflammatory demyelinating neuropathy remains in patients who do not meet the proposed electrodiagnostic criteria for demyelination. Nerve biopsy also has its pitfalls because the demyelinating process is not homogeneous and is basically asymmetrical, and because marked inflammatory infiltrates are not always present at the site of biopsy. Nerve biopsy may show only non-specific lesions when demyelination and inflammation are proximal to the site of the biopsy. Thus, each method has its limits.

Neuroimaging

An increased signal intensity on T2-weighted images of the brachial plexus can be seen on MRI in patients with CIDP, and also in patients with multifocal motor neuropathy (MMN), which may be useful to differentiate the latter from lower motor neuron disease. MRI study may show hypertrophy of spinal roots and plexuses with or without gadolinium enhancement. It is useful to know, however, that increased signal intensity on T2-weighted images of the brachial plexus and sciatic nerve can occur in other conditions including infiltrating malignant lymphoma and sciatica secondary to disk herniation, as we have observed.

Morphological findings

Peripheral nervous system (PNS) lesions consist of patchy regions of demyelination with variable inflammatory infiltrates, endoneurial oedema, demyelinated fibres, macrophage-mediated demyelination, remyelination, Schwann cell proliferation with onion-bulb formation, inflammatory infiltration with mononuclear cells, axonal degeneration, and axon loss (Figures 1 and 2). The presence of macrophage stripping of the myelin sheath is diagnostic of an inflammatory demyelinating neuropathy. However, the demonstration of macrophage stripping of the myelin sheath and even of inflammatory infiltrate is far from universal in nerve biopsy

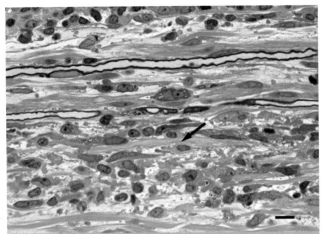

Figure 1. Longitudinal section of a nerve biopsy specimen from a patient with CIDP. The arrow points to a demyelinated axon surrounded by a number of mononuclear cells. (Bar: 10μm.)

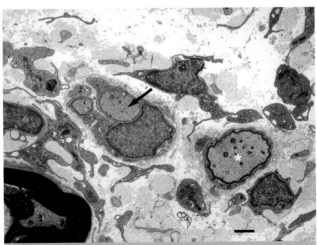

Figure 2. Electron micrograph of a cross-section of a nerve biopsy specimen from a patient with CIDP to show a demyelinated axon (arrow) and a remyelinating axon surrounded by a thin myelin sheath (asterisk). (Bar: 1μm.)

specimens. An important finding was that the density of myelinated nerve fibres was below 50% of control values in 47% of patients [3].

Immunological factors

Both cell-mediated mechanisms and an antibody-mediated response to major glycolipid or myelin protein antigens have been incriminated. CD4+ and CD8+ T-cells may be demonstrated in nerve biopsy specimens, but macrophages constitute the major cell component of the inflammatory infiltrate. Conflicting results have been reported recently with regard to the antibody-mediated mechanisms. In summary, an immune mechanism is very likely in CIDP but no reliable immunological test or diagnostic tool is available so far.

Differential diagnosis

A search for monoclonal gammopathy (monoclonal proliferation of lymphoid cells producing immunoglobulins) is important in patients with CIDP. Several patterns of demyelinating polyneuropathies can be associated with monoclonal gammopathy. The most common pattern is the association of CIDP with benign monoclonal gammopathy of unknown significance (MGUS).

The major difference between patients with MGUS and CIDP is the risk of malignancy in the following years in patients with MGUS and an acquired demyelinating polyneuropathy, so patients need to be periodically tested for this possibility.

The association of demyelinating polyneuropathy, organomegaly with endocrinopathy, monoclonal gammopathy and skin lesions is known as the POEMS syndrome. In this syndrome, progressive sensory-motor demyelinating polyneuropathy is associated with monoclonal gammopathy and other uncommon manifestations including skin pigmentation, hepatosplenomegaly, papilloedema, enlarged lymph nodes, endocrinopathy, oedema, thrombocytosis, and elevated vascular endothelial growth factor (VEGF). A total body scan must be performed to detect sclerotic bone lesions. This syndrome often responds well to specific treatment for plasmacytoma [10].

A life-threatening disorder results from the presence of light chain-derived amyloid deposits in the nerve endoneurium and other organs. In this setting, the occurrence of autonomic disturbances, in association with the monoclonal gammopathy, in a patient with progressive acquired demyelinating polyneuropathy suggests the development of light chain amyloid neuropathy. This has a very poor prognosis due to progressive axonal degeneration of the majority of the peripheral nerve fibres and multiorgan failure.

Treatment

Corticosteroids, IVIGs, plasma exchange and immunosuppressive drugs are the main treatments used in this condition [11]. Nearly all patients with CIDP will show an initial response to immunomodulatory therapy. Evaluation of response to treatment, however, is hampered by the lack of objective measures, poor correlation with electrophysiological data, variable incidence of axonal degeneration (which is unlikely to respond quickly to treatment) and the variability of the spontaneous course of the disease.

Prednisone is usually started and maintained at 1mg/kg/day for a few weeks and then tapered gently over several months. Alternatively, treatment can start with a high-dose IVIG (0.4g per kg body weight, on 5 consecutive days), then once a month for 3 months, although at lower doses; a total dose of 1g/kg body weight over 3 days did work in most of our cases. Where this fails, plasma exchange can be tried.

Other treatment with immunosuppressive drugs including cyclophosphamide, azathioprine, mycophenolate, and ciclosporin, has been tried in patients who did not respond to previous treatments, but the response is very variable. These drugs can be used as steroid-sparing agents. A number of questions remain unanswered regarding the pathophysiology, management and treatment of CIDP, which remains a disabling and sometimes life-threatening disorder.

➲ **Key points**

- The diagnosis of CIDP is based on the association of a proximal and distal motor deficit of subacute onset, nerve conduction slowing and increased CSF protein content.
- Sensory CIDP is difficult to diagnose without a nerve biopsy.
- The course of CIDP can be subacute progressive or relapsing.
- CIDP is often associated with monoclonal gammopathy of unknown significance.
- Corticosteroids, IVIGs and plasma exchange can be tried in CIDP.

References

1. Ad Hoc Subcommittee of the American Academy of Neurology AIDS Task Force. Research criteria for the diagnosis of chronic inflammatory demyelinating polyradiculoneuropathy (CIDP). *Neurology* 1991; 41: 617-8.

2. Said G, Krarup C. Chronic inflammatory demyelinative polyneuropathy. *Handb Clin Neurol* 2013; 115: 403-13.

3. Bouchard C, Lacroix C, Planté V, *et al*. Clinicopathological findings and prognosis of chronic inflammatory demyelinating polyneuropathy. *Neurology* 1999; 52: 498-503.

4. Dyck PJ, Lais AC, Ohta M, *et al*. Chronic inflammatory polyradiculoneuropathy. *Mayo Clinic Proc* 1975; 50: 621-37.

5. McCombe PA, Pollard JD, McLeod JG. Chronic inflammatory demyelinating polyradiculoneuropathy. *Brain* 1987; 110: 1617-30.

6. Gorson KC, Ropper AH, Weinberg DH. Upper limb predominant, multifocal chronic inflammatory demyelinating polyneuropathy. *Muscle Nerve* 1999; 22: 758-65.

7. Ferreira P, Lozeron C, Lacroix D, *et al*. Sensory chronic inflammatory demyelinating polyneuropathy: a study of 28 cases with nerve biopsy. *J Neurol* 2003; 250: 149.

8. Simmons Z, Albers JW, Bromberg M, Feldman EL. Long-term follow-up of patients with chronic inflammatory demyelinating polyradiculoneuropathy, without and with monoclonal gammopathy. *Brain* 1995; 48: 359-68.

9. Gorson KC, Ropper AH, Adelman LS, Weinberg DH. Influence of diabetes mellitus on chronic inflammatory demyelinating polyneuropathy. *Muscle Nerve* 2000; 23: 37-43.

10. Dispenzieri A. How I treat POEMS syndrome. *Blood* 2012; 119: 5650-8.

11. Lehmann HC, Hughes RA, Hartung HP. Treatment of chronic inflammatory demyelinating polyradiculoneuropathy. *Handb Clin Neurol* 2013; 115: 415-27.

Chapter 6

Vasculitic neuropathies

Overview

This chapter describes how an inflammation of blood vessels can cause neuropathies by affecting the blood vessels that supply nerves (vasa nervorum). These disorders can occur as part of connective tissue illness such as rheumatoid arthritis or in primary vasculitides. Occlusion of nerve blood vessels provokes ischaemia of nerve trunks and axonal degeneration of nerve fibres. Lesions predominate in nerve trunks of the limbs typically inducing a multifocal sensory and motor neuropathy. Systemic manifestations are often associated with nerve and skin lesions. Nerve biopsy is usually required to demonstrate lesions of nerve blood vessels. The mainstay of treatment is prednisolone, but recovery can be slow and relapses are frequent.

Introduction

Vasculitis occurs as a primary phenomenon in connective tissue disorders (CTDs) and associated illnesses, including polyarteritis nodosa (PAN) and the Churg-Strauss syndrome (CSS) variant, rheumatoid arthritis, systemic lupus erythematosus (SLE), and granulomatosis with polyangiitis (GP) [1]. In all these conditions focal and multifocal neuropathy occur as a consequence of nerve ischaemia related to destruction of the arterial wall and occlusion of the lumen of small epineurial arteries. Vasculitis may also complicate the course of other conditions ranging from infection with the human immunodeficiency virus (HIV) and with the B and C hepatitis viruses to diabetes and sarcoidosis. In all instances, symptomatic vasculitis requires corticosteroids to control the inflammatory process and prevent further ischaemic nerve lesions.

Pathophysiology of vasculitis

Primary vasculitis and connective tissue disorders

Primary vasculitides are often classified according to the size of vessels predominantly affected. In medium-sized vessels, vasculitic neuropathy occurs only in patients with PAN. The group of small-vessel vasculitic neuropathies includes GP, the CSS [2], and microscopic polyangiitis with capillary involvement.

The diagnosis of PAN is histological. Criteria include transmural infiltration of small arteries with polymorphonuclear cells (often admixed with lymphocytes and eosinophils), leukocytoclasia, fibrinoid necrosis, destruction of the internal elastic lamina, occlusion of the lumen and the usual sparing of adjacent venules (Figure 1).

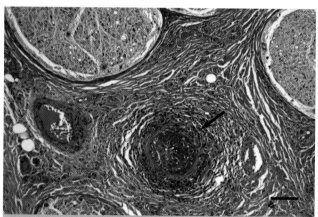

Figure 1. Nerve biopsy from a patient with multifocal neuropathy due to polyarteritis nodosa. Nerve cross-section of the paraffin-embedded specimen shows necrotizing arteritis of an epineurial artery (arrow). (Hematein eosin staining. Bar: 100μm.)

Granulomatosis with polyangiitis (GP) is an antibody-mediated autoimmune, granulomatous vasculitis, in which antibodies against proteinase 3 and myeloperoxidase are demonstratable in the serum of patients. Serologic demonstration of these anti-neutrophil cytoplasmic antibodies (ANCAs) is a sensitive and specific means by which to diagnose GP.

Secondary vasculitis

In vasculitis secondary to inflammatory and infectious disorders, the role of cellular factors is often prominent. In such conditions, macrophages and cytotoxic T-lymphocytes seem to play a major role in vessel wall damage.

The peripheral neuropathy of necrotizing arteritis (NA)

Typically, the clinical picture is that of an acute or subacute mononeuritis multiplex. However, distal symmetrical sensory or sensorimotor neuropathy occurs in 40% of cases. The peroneal nerve is the most commonly affected nerve unilaterally or bilaterally, whilst in the upper extremities, the ulnar nerve is the most commonly affected.

In typical cases, the onset of the neuropathy is abrupt and the deficit severe, but a partial deficit in a nerve territory is often observed. A slowly progressive course is frequently seen in the elderly.

Recovery from motor deficit due to ischaemic neuropathy takes months, because of the axonal pattern of nerve damage. Residual pain is common and may be difficult to differentiate from relapses of the neuropathy. Autonomic dysfunction is uncommon.

Electrophysiological studies (electromyography [EMG] and nerve conduction time [NCT]) show evidence of an axonal neuropathy.

Demonstration of NA in nerve and muscle biopsy specimens

The diagnosis of NA needs histological confirmation, which can sometimes be achieved by biopsying a specific skin lesion. If not, nerve and/or muscle biopsies can be obtained in the search for characteristic lesions of muscular or epineurial arteries. It is impossible to tell how often the diagnosis of NA cannot be achieved histologically. Not finding evidence of vasculitis in the nerve biopsy specimen does not rule out the diagnosis of NA as there is a general belief that the false-negative rate for biopsy is significant.

When characteristic lesions are not found on the first sections, serial sections of the biopsy specimens must be studied because NA is segmental, and characteristic lesions may be present over segments of the arteries as short as 50μm in our experience. The yield of a positive biopsy studied on serial sections increased by 36% for muscle specimens and by 53% for nerve specimens [3].

Lesions of nerve fibres — ischaemic neuropathy

Nerve ischaemia, as observed in vasculitic neuropathy, always induces acute axonal degeneration. Asymmetry of lesions between and within fascicles is also common in vasculitic neuropathy. Sometimes axon loss predominates in the centrofascicular area (middle of the nerve bundle), which is also suggestive of an ischaemic origin.

Clinical aspects

Classical polyarteritis nodosa

NA of the polyarteritis nodosa (PAN) type is the most homogeneous entity. NA occurs *de novo* in PAN, or as a secondary feature in diseases such as rheumatoid arthritis and, occasionally, in systemic lupus erythematosus. The consequences of vascular inflammation and occlusion depend on the size and number of blood vessels affected. Clinical neuropathy occurs in 50-75% of patients with systemic vasculitis of the PAN group.

In one of our studies we found that classic PAN affected 24% of our patients [3]. In these patients, multisystem involvement was present with cutaneous vasculitis as the most common non-neurological manifestation. Specific skin involvement includes livedo reticularis, cutaneous necrosis and nodules. Non-specific oedema, usually affecting one limb extremity, often precedes the onset of neuropathy. Renal involvement was observed in 9% and asthma in 7% of our patients.

Churg and Strauss variant of polyarteritis nodosa

Churg-Strauss syndrome applies to disseminated necrotising vasculitis occurring among asthmatic patients, with fever, eosinophilia, and a fulminant multisystem disease with a pathology of NA, eosinophilic infiltration and extravascular granulomas.

The vascular and nerve lesions observed in nerve biopsies from patients with this syndrome are similar to those observed in PAN. Perinuclear anti-neutrophil cytoplasmic antibodies (pANCAs) seem to be commonly found in this syndrome.

Necrotising arteritis and neuropathy in patients with rheumatoid arthritis (⊃ see case study overleaf)

The occurrence of NA in the context of rheumatoid arthritis is classically associated with a poor outcome. In our study of 32 patients with rheumatoid arthritis and neuropathy due to histologically proven necrotising vasculitis in muscle and/or nerve biopsy specimens, 15 had a sensory and motor neuropathy, the others a purely sensory neuropathy. Two thirds of the patients had a multifocal pattern of neurological deficit, the other third manifested distal symmetrical sensory neuropathy [4].

Vasculitic neuropathy associated with rheumatoid arthritis

Cheryl is a 43-year-old right-handed former lunchtime supervisor who presented with joint problems in her early thirties. She had been followed up in the rheumatology clinics and started developing painful and numb feet. She had initially been treated with non-steroidal anti-inflammatories, but for a number of years had been treated with intermittent courses of prednisolone and had also been treated with disease- modifying drugs including hydroxychloroquine and sulfasalazine. By the time she arrived at the neurology clinic she was taking 15mg of prednisolone a day and cyclophosphamide 1mg a day.

Examination revealed advanced rheumatoid changes in the joints of the hands and feet. Power was difficult to ascertain due to the joint deformity and pain, but was probably near normal. The sensory examination revealed a loss of pain perception to the wrists and 7cm above the ankles, with a similar loss of temperature perception. Vibration sensation was lost in the toes, but was present in the hands and ankles. Joint position sense was lost in her toes, but was present at the ankles, and normal in the hands. The deep tendon reflexes were generally diminished and lost at the ankles. The plantar responses were difficult to interpret and her gait was wide-based and unsteady.

She was regularly reviewed in the neurology clinic and the waxing and waning of her neuropathy, together with her inflammatory markers and rheumatological examination, informed her rheumatologist, as to the dose of steroid and changes in her disease-modifying antirheumatic drugs.

Granulomatosis with polyangiitis

Granulomatosis with polyangiitis (GP) is characterised by granulomatous vasculitis of the upper and lower respiratory tract with or without glomerulonephritis. Peripheral neuropathy has been observed in 25% of patients with GP [5]. Peripheral neuropathy seldom is the first manifestation of the disease. In a review of 324 patients with GP, 109 had neurological manifestations at some stage. Fifty-three patients had peripheral neuropathy, which was multifocal in 42. Cranial nerves were involved in 21/109, ophthalmoplegia in 16/21. The mean interval between the onset of GP and neurological manifestations was 8.4 months [5].

Necrotising arteritis and isolated neuropathy

In a large proportion of patients with peripheral neuropathy related to necrotising arteritis seen in neurology, there is no organ clinically involved other than the peripheral nervous system (PNS) [6]. This group of patients accounted for 21% of patients seen with demonstrated NA and neuropathy in our service. In such patients peripheral neuropathy is the presenting and only manifestation of necrotising arteritis.

Silent involvement of other organs is common in such patients, however, as shown by the frequent finding of necrotising arteritis in muscle biopsy specimens. Thus, it seems more appropriate to consider that patients with apparently isolated vasculitic neuropathy are affected by a low-grade vasculitis, symptomatic in nerves only, because tissue ischaemia is more likely to be symptomatic in nerves than in most other organs.

From a neurological standpoint, approximately one fourth of patients presented with a distal symmetrical sensory or sensorimotor neuropathy, and the diagnosis of NA had seldom been considered before the results of the nerve and muscle biopsies. During follow-up, one third of the patients in this group developed systemic manifestations. A relapse of the neuropathy occurred in 25% of patients.

Vasculitic neuropathy in the elderly

Neuropathy is an important factor of disability in the elderly. In a series of 100 patients over 65 years of age referred for a disabling neuropathy, we found that 23% had vasculitic neuropathy with necrotising vasculitis demonstrated in the nerve and/or muscle biopsy specimen(s). Most patients responded well to treatment. In this group of patients, the neuropathy occurred in the context of a multisystem disorder in two thirds of patients, and as an isolated neuropathy in 10 patients [7].

Secondary vasculitic neuropathy

Vasculitis can complicate the course of different conditions including an inflammatory immune reaction triggered by an infective agent, a delayed-type hypersensitivity reaction, diabetes mellitus or malignancy.

Necrotising vasculitis and viral infection

Symptomatic viral infection, including HIV infection, opportunistic infection with cytomegalovirus at a late stage of HIV infection, chronic hepatitis B and C viruses, and human T-lymphotropic virus type I (HTLV-1) infection can be associated with neuropathy and necrotising vasculitis. The clinical pattern of vasculitic neuropathy observed in association with hepatitis B and C viral infection is similar to that of primary vasculitis. In this setting the neuropathy can also be associated with cryoglobulinaemia, which occurs in patients with malignant gammopathy as well.

Sarcoidosis

The occurrence of necrotising vasculitis in association with granuloma secondary to the delayed hypersensitivity reaction that characterises sarcoidosis, stresses the need to exclude other causes of granulomatous angiitis, especially GP, which differs from sarcoidosis both clinically and biologically.

Vasculitis in diabetic neuropathy

Inflammatory lesions of nerve blood vessels play a role in focal and multifocal diabetic neuropathy. (Please refer to Chapter 8 — Diabetic and uraemic neuropathies — for more detail.)

Vasculitis in malignancy

Paraneoplastic neuropathies are sometimes associated with vasculitis.

(Please refer to Chapter 9 — Neuropathies in patients with monoclonal gammopathy and malignancy — for more detail.)

Treatment

Treatment is based on administration of corticosteroids and immunosuppressive drugs. Prednisone should be started at 1mg/kg/day. Simultaneous treatment with cyclophosphamide, 2mg/kg/day, may help to reduce the dose of corticosteroids. In cases with severe general manifestations, pulses of intravenous prednisolone may help. It is difficult to stipulate how long this treatment should be maintained at full dose. This depends on the response to treatment, on the course and form of the disease, and on the tolerance of the treatment. A full steroid dose is usually given for approximately 6-8 weeks and is subsequently tapered over a period of 6-10 months or more. It is necessary to control the erythrocyte sedimentation rate (ESR) and other markers of disease activity including C-reactive protein (CRP) and eosinophilic polymorphonuclear cell levels, which may vary from one patient to another, and to adjust the doses of prednisone accordingly. Many patients relapse either during reduction of steroid therapy or after treatment has been stopped. In our experience, up to half of patients relapse during tapering of prednisone or after treatment has been stopped. Careful follow-up of patients is mandatory.

In cases without clinical evidence of polysystemic involvement, or with a normal ESR, and in elderly patients, the benefit of prolonged treatment with high doses of steroids is less certain. Indomethacin (100mg/day) may be added to steroids when fever persists or when the ESR remains abnormal in spite of large doses of steroids.

Whilst evaluating the efficacy of the treatment of vasculitic neuropathies, it must be remembered that there is a wide range of evolving modalities in NA, and that spontaneous remission of several years' duration can occur. Sensorimotor deficit resulting from nerve ischaemia will take months to recover, because of the underlying axonal lesions. Motor recovery will be helped by physiotherapy, but residual pain is common.

➡ Key points

- Vasculitic neuropathy is typically a multifocal painful, motor and sensory neuropathy of subacute onset.
- Inflammation and necrosis of nerve blood vessels cause ischaemic nerve lesions.
- Vasculitis can be primary as in polyarteritis nodosa or secondary to systemic disorders.
- Nerve and muscle biopsies are needed for diagnosis in most cases.
- In a large proportion of patients neuropathy is the only manifestation of vasculitis.
- Treatment rests on corticosteroid and immunosuppressive drugs.

References

1. Falk RJ, Gross WL, Guillevin L, et al. Rheumatism. Granulomatosis with polyangiitis (Wegener's): an alternative name for Wegener's granulomatosis. Arthritis Rheum 2011; 63: 863-4.

2. Churg J, Strauss L. Allergic granulomatosis, allergic angiitis, and periarteritis nodosa. Am J Pathol 1951; 27: 277-301.

3. Said G, Lacroix C, Fujimura H, et al. The peripheral neuropathy of necrotizing arteritis: a clinicopathologic study. Ann Neurol 1988; 23: 461-5.

4. Vrancken AF, Said G. Vasculitic neuropathy. Handb Clin Neurol 2013; 115: 463-83.

5. Nishino H, Rubino FA, DeRemee RA, et al. Neurological involvement in Wegener's granulomatosis: an analysis of 324 consecutive patients at the Mayo Clinic. Ann Neurol 1993; 33: 4-9.

6. Dyck PJ, Benstead TJ, Conn DL, et al. Nonsystemic vasculitic neuropathy. Brain 1987; 110: 843-54.

7. Chia L, Fernandez A, Lacroix C, et al. Contribution of nerve biopsy findings to the diagnosis of disabling neuropathy in the elderly: a retrospective review of 100 consecutive patients. Brain 1996; 119: 1091-8.

Chapter 7

Infectious neuropathies

Overview

This chapter deals with the different infective processes that may affect the peripheral nervous system. Leprous neuropathy, with its two patterns — lepromatous and tuberculoid — still affects several million people, mainly in intertropical developing countries. *Mycobacterium leprae* is predominantly found in nerve trunks and skin. Lyme disease due to infection by *Borrelia burgdorferi* is transmitted by a tick bite. It induces a benign meningoradiculitis lasting a few weeks. HIV infection can induce a variety of peripheral neuropathies plus cytomegalovirus neuropathy that occurs at the end stage of HIV infection.

Introduction

Inflammatory neuropathies can be defined as neuropathies in which lesions of peripheral nerve fibres are associated with inflammatory infiltration. In most instances, inflammatory neuropathies follow infection of the peripheral nervous system by viruses, bacteria or parasites. This group is the largest group of neuropathies in the world. In this context nerve lesions can result from the inflammatory reaction induced by the infective agent or from the immune reaction of the patient.

Leprosy

Leprous neuropathy, which is due to infection of nerve cells by *Mycobacterium leprae*, still affects millions of people in many developing countries. The clinical and pathological manifestations are determined by the natural resistance of the host to invasion of *Mycobacterium leprae*. Failure of early detection of leprosy often leads to severe disability in spite of eradication of mycobacteria at a later date. In the lepromatous type, bacilli are easily found in the skin, and in nerve cells including Schwann cells, endothelial cells and macrophages (Figure 1). In the tuberculoid type, a strong cell-mediated immune reaction leads to granuloma formation and destruction of cells harbouring bacilli and neighbouring nerve fibres. In many cases treatment of patients with multibacillary leprosy is complicated by reversal reaction and further nerve damage (Figures 2 and 3) [1, 2].

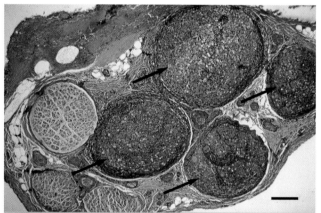

Figure 1. Nerve biopsy from a patient with lepromatous leprous neuropathy to show partial involvement of a nerve trunk. Four fascicles (arrows) are affected while the other three appear normal at this magnification. (Bar: 1mm.)

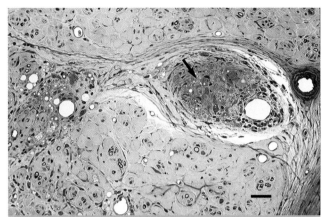

Figure 2. Nerve biopsy from a patient with a late upgrade reversal reaction that occurred more than 20 years after treatment of a multibacillary leprous neuropathy. Note the granulomas close to an epineurial blood vessel (arrow). The endoneurium is filled with connective tissue with a few regenerating nerve fibres. (One-micron-thick plastic section. Toluidine blue staining. Bar: 50μm.)

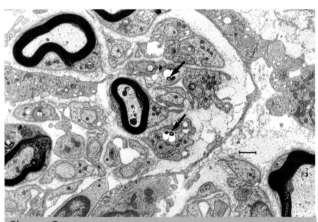

Figure 3. Electron micrograph of a nerve biopsy specimen from a patient with lepromatous (multibacillary) leprous neuropathy at an early stage. Note the preservation of many myelinated and unmyelinated nerve fibres. Bacilli can be seen in vacuoles in the cytoplasm of some Schwann cells (arrows). (Uranyl acetate and lead citrate staining. Bar: 1μm.)

Historical and epidemiological aspects

Leprosy has been recognised since the ancient civilisations of China, Egypt and India. The oldest description of leprosy probably dates back to 600 B.C. At that time it used to be considered a divine punishment for sins, according to the Old Testament, and to karma in the Buddhist religion. In 1874, Hansen identified the causal agent of this illness at a time when leprosy was endemic in Norway [3].

Subsequent improvements in the treatment, management and public health approach have contributed to a near eradication of the disease in industrialised countries. Yet leprosy still remains among the first causes for neuropathy in the world even though the latest estimate of the number of leprosy cases worldwide is 5.5 million (which is about half the number estimated in the early 1980s), with 2-3 million patients having residual deformity.

Leprosy is primarily found in tropical and sub-tropical developing countries, with some parts of Asia and Africa having a prevalence exceeding 10 per 1000 population and more than 0.5 million new cases detected each year. During 2008, 17 countries reported more than 1000 new cases. Leprosy continues to be an important health problem worldwide but is most prevalent in India, Brazil, Indonesia and Nigeria. India accounts for 64% of worldwide cases [4].

Pathophysiology

Several features of leprosy are unique and strikingly different from other infectious diseases of man, in relation to the nature of the infective agent and to the immunological status of the host. Much of the neurological aspects of leprous neuropathies has been known for decades, yet leprosy remains a subject of interest because the form of leprosy mainly depends on the immune reaction of the host to *Mycobacterium leprae* antigens, ranging in extremes from the lowest cell-mediated immunity to *Mycobacterium leprae*, the lepromatous pole, to that of the highest immune response, the tuberculoid pole.

Mycobacterium leprae

Leprosy is caused by *Mycobacterium leprae*, an intracellular gram-positive alcohol-acid-fast bacillus. It is morphologically indistinguishable from *Mycobacterium tuberculosis*. It doesn't grow in human temperatures at 37°C; the optimal temperature for growth is between 27-30°C. This accounts for the predominance of leprous lesions in the coldest areas of the body.

Mycobacterium leprae is an obligatory intracellular parasite with tropism for macrophages and Schwann cells. This preference is determined by the attachment of the bacterium onto the alfa-2 chain 'G' unit found in the basal lamina of Schwann cells. This lamina is only found in peripheral nerves. At any given moment, T-cells will recognise the bacterium inside and hence trigger a subacute and later chronic inflammatory response. This results in progressive damage to both myelinated and unmyelinated nerve fibres followed by replacement of functional tissue by conjunctive tissue. The phenolic glycolipid-1 (PGL-1) is a cell-wall antigen on the surface of *Mycobacterium leprae* through which it attaches to Schwann cells. Nerve fibrosis is responsible for irreversible nerve damage in leprous neuropathy.

Transmission

Both nasal secretions and skin from untreated multibacillary cases of leprosy are capable of shedding *Mycobacterium leprae* to the environment, which may be deposited on either or both the nasal and skin epithelia when in contact with others and so potentially initiating infection. Haematogenous dissemination is widely accepted as the most likely route of infection in the lepromatous form. The incubation period is extremely variable. It may be as long as 10-20 years. Exposure to the bacillus is not sufficient for the disease to develop. Factors such as nutrition, hygiene and house crowding play an important role. There is a male preponderance in the lepromatous form and a female excess in the tuberculoid type.

Clinical manifestations

Specific cutaneous lesions

Specific cutaneous lesions, including maculae and lepromae, reveal the disease in half or more of patients, depending on the type of leprosy. In others, small areas of sensory loss, limited anhydrosis and alopecia zones, paresis of facial muscles, hypochromic or atrophic cutaneous zones or painful enlargement of a nerve trunk are the presenting manifestations. Plantar ulcers and other trophic changes occur later in the course of the disease, as a consequence of sensory loss.

Sensory loss

Sensory loss is the most constant finding of leprous neuropathy. Sensory loss, which is due to mixed dermal nerve and nerve trunk damage, is extremely variable in distribution, ranging from a small skin patch with impaired sensation to severe sensory loss over most of the body surface, but avoiding the body folds. Early cutaneous lesions show some preservation of sensation, with impairment of light touch, and loss of thermal and pain sense, which leads to painless trauma and trophic changes. Proprioception is preserved, so patients can still use their largely anaesthetic limbs effectively. Loss of dermal pigment in the territory of affected cutaneous nerves leads to the development of large anaesthetic patches in dark-skinned people, with loss of sweating in corresponding areas. Colder areas of the body seem more affected, but temperature-linked sensory loss, which is not observed in tuberculoid leprosy, cannot account for all patterns of nerve lesions in leprosy. In some cases, complete loss of pain and temperature sensation in a certain area contrasts with preservation of tactile sensation. This classical dissociation of sensory loss is seldom complete in leprosy. In most cases all modalities of superficial sensation are affected. Sensory loss also occurs in the areas corresponding to maculae, demonstrating early involvement of sensory nerve terminals.

The topographical distribution of sensory disturbance is extremely variable. Sensory loss may form an 'insular' pattern, in which anaesthetic areas of variable forms, size and number are found, and these areas may or may not correlate with the macular-type cutaneous lesions. This sensory loss, which may last for years, is usually associated with other disturbances such as anhydrosis, alopecia and vasomotor areflexia. These manifestations are related to lesions of sensory nerve endings or to that of a limited number of nerve fascicles of a nerve trunk. Sensory loss may also display a nerve trunk pattern. In cases of longstanding evolution, the distal part of the limbs show the greatest sensory loss. This extends proximally to a greater or lesser extent, rarely to the trunk. When the trunk is involved, sensory loss affects an insular pattern. This pattern of sensory loss does not affect the anterior aspect of the trunk in a length-dependent pattern, as in severe diabetic, amyloid or alcoholic polyneuropathy. In individual patients, dissociation between sensations may be found in some areas only. The large nerve trunks most commonly affected are the ulnar and the lateral popliteal nerves, followed by the median, posterior tibial, superficial radial, peroneal nerves, and the greater auricular and facial nerves.

Nerve hypertrophy

Nerve trunks are palpably enlarged in one third of patients with leprosy, sometimes before the occurrence of sensory loss in the corresponding territory [5]. Superficial nerves like the greater auricular nerve in the neck, the supraorbitary branch of the trigeminal nerve or larger nerve trunks, especially the ulnar nerve above the elbow, the peroneal nerve, and the radial cutaneous nerve at the lateral border of the wrist, are often enlarged.

Motor disturbance and amyotrophy

Motor involvement is usually a late event in the course of the disease. Amyotrophy and motor weakness usually progress equally; in some cases, however, amyotrophy is more marked than weakness, which both predominate in the ulnar and median nerve territories, with characteristic claw hands. Preservation of deep tendon reflexes in many cases of leprous neuropathy is characteristic of the predominant involvement of the most distal part of the nerves.

Facial palsy

Facial palsy with lagophthalmos of one or both eyes, with sparing of the other muscles supplied by the facial nerve, is a classical feature of leprosy.

Trophic disturbances

Trophic plantar ulcers are a common, non-specific complication of loss of pain sensation over the plantar sole. Severe sensory disturbances are always found in those areas where ulcers occur. Plantar ulcers occur subsequent to microtrauma on skin that has lost painful sensation. The absence of protective sensation in limb extremities leads to overuse, accidental self-injury, recurrent infections, and to a gradual development of further deformities as observed in sensory neuropathy of a different origin.

The spectrum of clinical manifestations correlates well with the cellular immune responsiveness of the patient to *Mycobacterium leprae* antigens, which range from the lowest cell-mediated immunity to *Mycobacterium leprae*, the lepromatous pole, to that of the highest cell-mediated immunity, the tuberculoid pole [6].

Different patterns of leprous neuropathy

Two main patterns of leprous neuropathy have been identified: the lepromatous type or multibacillary leprous neuropathy, and the tuberculoid leprous neuropathy or paucibacillary leprous neuropathy [7-9].

Lepromatous and borderline lepromatous leprosy — multibacillary leprosy

These represent the most common types of leprosy in many endemic areas of Africa. In nearly all cases they are associated with characteristic skin lesions. Occasionally, there is no detectable skin lesion. Skin lesions, however, are usually numerous consisting of macules, papules and nodules with infiltration and thickening of the skin, affecting predominantly the cooler areas of the body. At this stage, diffuse, bilateral and generally symmetrical nerve damage occurs. In such patients bacteria can be found in skin lesions, nasal smears, or even in blood with a majority of circulating bacilli found intracellularly, in polymorphonuclear leukocytes, monocytes and large circulating histiocytes.

In this form, the specific unresponsiveness of the host to antigens of the leprosy bacillus permits unchecked proliferation of bacilli.

Light microscopic examination of nerve cross-sections of affected nerves show an enormous inflammatory reaction affecting the epineurium of all nerve specimens and the perineurium of most fascicles [10]. This inflammatory reaction is responsible for the nerve enlargement. *Mycobacterium leprae* are extremely numerous, in all forms of lepromatous neuropathy; they are often in a globus arrangement, on Ziehl-stained paraffin-embedded specimens. *Mycobacterium leprae* are easily identified on electron microscopic examination as dark, osmiophilic spheres usually located in a cytoplasmic vacuole containing phenolic glycolipid-I (PGL-I) and lipoarabinomannan, both produced in large amounts by *Mycobacterium leprae.*

Another salient feature observed in nerves of patients with lepromatous leprosy is the intense proliferation of fibroblasts with increased synthesis of collagen, leading to endo- and peri-neurial fibrosis which can hamper growth of regenerating fibres. Control of unwanted sclerosis can certainly improve the outcome of the neuropathy.

Tuberculoid leprosy

At the other end of the spectrum, tuberculoid leprosy is identified by complete nerve destruction. In this form patients develop high levels of specific cell-mediated immunity that ultimately kills and clears the bacilli in the tissues, inducing simultaneous damage to the nerves that harbour the bacilli. Clinically, tuberculoid lesions may be single or few, and are distributed asymmetrically in the vicinity of typical hypoaesthetic or anaesthetic hypopigmented skin lesions. There is considerable evidence suggesting that patients with tuberculoid leprosy have nerve damage caused not by the bacilli but by the cell-mediated immune response to *Mycobacterium leprae* antigens.

Histopathologically, the lesion is characterised by epithelioid-cell granulomata with intense lymphocytic infiltration. Normal nerve structure may no longer be identified in many cases and bacilli are not found in the lesions, but *Mycobacterium leprae* antigens have been detected in nerves using anti-BCG (bacillus Calmette-Guérin) anti-sera which cross-react with *Mycobacterium leprae* antigens. In skin lesions the tuberculoid infiltrates predominantly contain helper T-cells. The basis for the conspicuous destruction of nerve structure is thought to be a delayed-type hypersensitivity reaction with specific helper T-cells reacting with *Mycobacterium leprae* antigens presented in the endoneurium by macrophages and possibly by Schwann cells expressing the HLA-DR antigen induced by interferon released by helper T-cells. Activation of macrophages in this context leads to the release of a number of secretory products noxious to surrounding cells.

Reactional states

One of the many concerns in patients under treatment for leprous neuropathy is the occurrence of a sudden alteration in immunological status and the development of a reactional state.

The reversal or upgrade form or type 1 reaction
This appears commonly during the first year of therapy, or up to decades later. It is characterised by a heightened cell-mediated response occurring mainly in patients with the borderline-lepromatous form of leprosy (⬤ see case study overleaf). This reaction is identified by swelling and exacerbation of existing skin and nerve lesions in association with general malaise and fever. Painful swelling of nerve trunks is accompanied by sensory and motor deficit in the corresponding territory. In some cases, nerves which were apparently unaffected are heavily damaged. Endoneurial granulomas, multinucleated giant cells, lymphocytic infiltration, vasculitis and perineuritis are present on morphological examination. Necrosis of the endoneurial content may lead to nerve abscesses. No *Mycobacterium leprae* are observed in this reaction.

Erythema nodosum leprosum (ENL)-type 2 reaction
ENL corresponds to a downgrade reaction. It is almost exclusively seen in the lepromatous pole in endemic areas. It is a complex systemic disorder affecting multiple organs. The appearance of typical erythematous skin lesions is the diagnostic criterion for ENL. Nodules and painful, raised, red papules are characteristic. Accompanying these nodules are uveitis, iridocyclitis, episcleritis, neuritis, arthritis, dactilitis, lymphoadenitis, and orchitis. Fever, prostration, anorexia, as well as other constitutional symptoms, are frequent, with the finding of chronic or sub-acute inflammatory infiltrates and areas of conjunctive tissue with or without bacilli.

Late reversal reaction in a patient with lepromatous leprous neuropathy

Peter was first seen at the age of 38. He was a school teacher living in French Polynesia. He was on a summer vacation in Europe and decided to consult for numbness in the hands. He was in good general condition. Hand numbness had started gradually on one side and subsequently affected both sides approximately 3 years before referral. Upon examination the patient had not noticed a loss of temperature, pain and light touch sensation over the lower extremities, up to the mid-leg. In the upper limbs sensory loss extended up to the elbows. Proprioception was preserved. Muscle strength and tendon reflexes were normal. The superficial radial nerve was enlarged and firm upon palpation. There were no skin lesions. A biopsy of the superficial radial nerve revealed multibacillar leprosy. The patient was put on a treatment regimen of rifampicin and dapsone for more than 2 years. His neurological condition improved although he retained some sensory loss 4 years later.

Six years after the diagnosis and start of the treatment, the patient experienced rapid worsening of his neurological condition with pains in all four limbs and walking difficulty. He had some fever and arthralgia. He had bilateral weakness of foot dorsiflexion and loss of sensation over both legs. A biopsy of the superficial peroneal nerve was performed. It showed loss of axons associated with endoneurial granulomas without any detectable *Mycobacterium leprae*. The patient's condition improved quickly after treatment with corticosteroids.

This patient had a late reversal reaction after treatment of lepromatous leprous neuropathy.

Diagnosis

The three diagnostic signs of leprosy are hypopigmented skin lesions with loss of sensation, thickening of peripheral nerves and skin-smear positivity for the acid-fast bacilli. In purely neuropathic forms which are seen in the tuberculoid form and, less often, in lepromatous leprosy, nerve biopsy is the only way to reach a diagnosis. It is especially useful in countries where leprosy is not common. In such countries, it must be noted that leprous neuropathy may become symptomatic years or decades after the patient has moved from endemic areas. In countries where leprosy is endemic, nerve biopsy may be useful in differentiating leprous neuropathy from a neuropathy of other origins, including diabetic neuropathy, hereditary sensory neuropathies or amyloid neuropathy which can lead to sensory and trophic manifestations that may be mistaken for leprous neuropathy. Ziehl's staining of paraffin-embedded sections permits visualisation of bacilli in the pluribacillar forms of the disease. Bacilli are scarce or absent from nerves with tuberculoid leprosy and in reversal reaction.

Treatment

In multibacillary leprosy, the standard treatment regimen is rifampicin 600mg once a month, dapsone 100mg daily, and clofazimine 300mg once a month and 50mg daily for 12 months, although in some patients treatment with these drugs may become necessary for up 24 months. In paucibacillary leprosy, the standard regimen is rifampicin 600mg once a month and dapsone 100mg daily for 6 months. Moreover, these regimens show a high frequency of reactional states both during and after treatment.

Patients who develop delayed nerve impairment months or years after treatment, which cannot be explained by relapses, must be treated with a more aggressive schedule of corticosteroids (higher dose and long duration).

Lyme disease

Lyme disease is a multisystem illness that affects the skin, joints, heart and nervous system, caused by a tick-transmitted spirochaete, *Borrelia burgdorferi*. The first description of tick-bite-associated paralysis and meningitis appeared in Europe [11-13], but the recognition of Lyme disease as a separate entity was made by Steere *et al* in 1977 in Lyme,

Connecticut (USA) [14]. Certain differences have been noted between American and European isolates of *Borrelia burgdorferi* in morphology, outer surface proteins, plasmids and DNA homology, which may account also for some clinical differences [15].

Ixodic ticks are the usual vectors. Ticks feed once during the three stages of their usual two-year life. Larval ticks take one blood meal in late summer, nymphs feed during the following spring and early summer, and adults during that autumn. In the United States, the preferred host for both the larval and nymphal stages is the white-footed mouse, while white-tailed deer are the preferred host of adult ixodes. In Europe, thousands of new cases occur each summer, particularly in central and northern Europe. In the United States, Lyme borreliosis is mainly reported from three areas: the Northeast, Midwest, and in California and Oregon in the West.

Clinical manifestations

The course of the disease follows three stages as outlined below.

Stage 1
The typical patient first has erythema migrans, sometimes followed several weeks or months later by meningitis or facial palsy, and often, months later by arthritis. Localised erythema migrans results from local spreading of *Borrelia burgdorferi* in the skin. It starts as a red macule or papule at the site of the bite and expands to form a large red ring with central clearing. It is accompanied by fever, minor constitutional symptoms, or regional lymphadenopathy.

Stage 2
Within days or weeks after inoculation, the spirochaete may spread in the patient's blood to many sites; spirochaetes have been recovered from blood during this stage and from many organs. Secondary annular lesions, which resemble the primary erythema migrans occur in about half of patients in association with migratory musculoskeletal and joint pain [16]. Widely disseminated symptoms seem to be more common in the United States than in Europe. By this time, the host starts to develop a strong

immune response to *Borrelia burgdorferi* antigens that result in destruction of spirochaetes by complement activation through immune complexes.

After several weeks or months, 15-20% of patients develop neurologic signs, often radicular pain of a burning type, which may or may not be associated with weakness, and with little or no clinical signs of meningitis (➲ see case study below). Painful meningoradiculitis is often called the

Lyme disease

John, a 59-year-old patient, had been treated with insulin for 10 years for type 1 diabetes, which had remained uncomplicated so far. At the end of May 2002 he started to complain of spontaneous burning pains in the right leg and inner and plantar aspects of the foot. Pain was present day and night, preventing sleep. Within a few days, pain extended over the dorsal aspect of the foot and the patient noticed some walking difficulty due to weakness of the right foot. Examination showed a sensory loss of pain, light touch, temperature and pinprick sensation over the dorsal and plantar aspects of the right foot and minimal weakness of foot dorsiflexion on the same side. The ankle jerk was abolished. There was no other clinical abnormality. The patient was in a good general condition. Electrophysiological examination showed that the sural nerve action potential was abolished on the right side and normal on the left side (10.93μV) with a normal nerve conduction velocity (40m/s).

A biopsy of the right superficial peroneal nerve revealed inflammatory infiltrates made up of mononuclear cells associated with axonal degeneration (Figure 4). Cerebrospinal fluid (CSF) examination showed pleocytosis at 15 cells/ml with a mixture of lymphocytes, polymorphonuclear cells, monocytes and macrophages. The protein level was 0.56g/L with oligoclonal bands.

After these findings of inflammatory nerve lesions and pleocytosis of the CSF, Lyme disease was queried and the patient was then questioned about tick bites. He revealed that he had had several tick bites months before without secondary erythema. Serological tests for *Borrelia burgdorferi* were positive in the blood and in the CSF. The patient recovered completely after treatment with ceftriaxone.

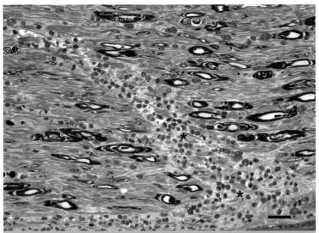

Figure 4. One-micron-thick plastic section of a biopsy specimen of the superficial peroneal nerve from a patient who presented with mononeuritis related to Lyme disease. Note the massive inflammatory infiltration (asterisks) and axonal degeneration of nerve fibres. (Toluidine blue staining. Bar: 20μm.)

Bannwarth's syndrome. Meningitis is the most common neurological abnormality in Lyme disease. It can be the first symptom of Lyme disease, but is preceded in most cases by erythema migrans, then usually begins after the skin lesions resolve. Papilloedema and increased cerebrospinal fluid (CSF) pressure can occur. CSF examination reveals a lymphocytic pleocytosis, usually a few tens or hundreds of cells per ml, with a mild elevation of protein with a high proportion of immunoglobulins and oligoclonal bands. The CSF glucose is usually normal but can be low. Spirochaetes have been cultured from CSF on several occasions.

Multifocal spinal root or cranial nerve involvement often develops within a few days or weeks, with uni- or bilateral facial palsy and asymmetric sensorimotor radiculoneuropathy. Cranial neuropathy is present in 50% of patients with neurological abnormalities. Facial palsy is often bilateral. Other cranial nerves can be affected, in association with meningitis. Cranial nerve palsies resolve within weeks or months, sometimes incompletely. Urinary and anal sphincter disturbance may also occur.

Peripheral neuropathy occurs in approximately half of patients with meningitis. Focal or multifocal involvement is the most common presentation. Common patterns include painful thoracoabdominal sensory radiculitis, associated with distal involvement. Both weakness and sensory loss improve within a few weeks, but recovery may take up to several months and often remains incomplete [17].

Electrophysiological testing of patients with peripheral neuropathy has shown evidence both of demyelination and of axonal degeneration, but usually axonal lesions predominate. Histologically, the nerve lesions are associated with lymphoplasmocytic inflammatory infiltrates that predominate in the nerve roots. The presence of *Borrelia burgdorferi* has not been convincingly documented in the nerves.

Cardiac involvement occurs in 4-8% of patients. They include fluctuating atrioventricular node block, mild left ventricular dysfunction, or, rarely, cardiomegaly or fatal pancarditis. The duration of cardiac abnormality is usually brief and does not necessitate the permanent insertion of a pacemaker [18].

Stage 3
Arthritis occurs in transient episodes, a mean of 6 months after the onset of the disease. Such episodes affect around 60% of patients in the United States and are characterised by asymmetric oligoarticular arthritis especially in the knee; one or a few joints may be affected. Spirochaetes have been occasionally cultured from joint fluid. Arthritis seems less common in Europe.

A variety of late syndromes affecting the central nervous system have been described, including spastic paraparesis, ataxia, relapsing multiple sclerosis-like illness, bladder dysfunction, cognitive impairment, dementia, and subacute encephalitis. Although these patients had serological evidence of Lyme disease, they did not have intrathecal synthesis of antibody to *Borrelia burgdorferi*. Thus, there is no convincing evidence for central nervous system complications of Lyme disease.

Diagnosis

From a neurological point of view, the presence of a subacute meningoradiculoneuritis with facial palsy and signs and symptoms suggesting a multifocal involvement of the peripheral nervous system, is highly suggestive of Lyme borreliosis. Serology is the only practical laboratory aid in diagnosis, but serologic testing is not yet standardised and the results from different laboratories may vary. The physician must be aware of false-negative and, more commonly, false-positive results [16]. Titres should increase four-fold or more between the erythema migrans phase and subsequent neurological involvement. Many patients have asymptomatic *Borrelia burgdorferi* infection, and equally, a false-positive result can occur, particularly with immunoglobulin M (IgM), both in healthy subjects and in patients with a variety of other diseases. Refinements of serologic methods may be helpful in the future to differentiate patients with residual positivity and a false-positive result from those suffering with Lyme disease.

Treatment

It must be kept in mind that Lyme disease is a benign condition. In a follow-up study of 72 patients up to 27 years after untreated Lyme neuroborreliosis, none of the patients showed signs of active disease or disease progression to chronic Lyme neuroborreliosis [19]. Treatment with high doses of penicillin gives good results at stage 1, but the results are not as good in patients with stage 2 neurologic abnormalities, and in patients with arthritis. *Borrelia burgdorferi* seems highly sensitive to tetracycline, ampicillin, ceftriaxone, but only moderately to penicillin. For early Lyme disease, localised stage 1 or disseminated stage 2 infection, oral tetracycline is generally an effective antibiotic [20]. Doxycycline, a long-acting tetracycline that achieves better tissue levels, may be preferable. The treatment should be administered for 10-30 days. The recommended dosage for 14 days is i.v. penicillin 20 million U daily in divided doses, cephalosporin, e.g. i.v. ceftriaxone 2g once a day, or oral doxycycline 100mg twice daily. Dose finding trials regarding the duration of treatment have never been conducted. In view of the low risk of Lyme disease after a recognised deer-tick bite and the uncertain effectiveness of prophylactic antimicrobial agents, routine antimicrobial prophylaxis for persons with a recognised deer-tick bite is not indicated.

Infection with retroviruses

Peripheral nerve lesions are commonly associated with human retroviral infection, which includes infection with the human immunodeficiency virus (HIV), the causal agent of AIDS, and, less commonly, the human T-lymphotropic virus type I (HTLV-1), the causal agent of tropical myeloneuropathy.

Neuropathies in HIV infection

Although the annual number of new HIV infections has been steadily declining since the late 1990s, this decrease is offset by the reduction in AIDS-related deaths due to the significant improvements in antiretroviral therapy (ART) over the past few years. Highly active antiretroviral therapy (HAART) and combined antiretroviral therapy (cART) have enabled sustained suppression of HIV replication and recovery of CD4+ T-cell counts; however, there is still no cure for HIV infection on the horizon [21, 22].

Symptomatic neuropathy affects an estimated 5-10% of HIV-infected patients. A wide variety of neuropathies have been observed in the course of HIV infection, and in some cases, neuropathy can be the first and only manifestation of HIV infection. The neuropathies observed in HIV patients include inflammatory polyneuropathy of the Guillain-Barré type, multifocal neuropathy, meningoradiculoneuritis, acute uni- or bilateral facial palsy and pandysautonomia. All these manifestations can be associated with central nervous system involvement or with inflammatory myopathy [23].

Inflammatory polyneuritis of the Guillain-Barré type

Guillain-Barré syndrome (GBS) can be observed at the time of seroconversion to HIV. Mild to severe motor deficit is associated with high fever, diarrhoea, rash, adenopathy and mononucleosic syndrome. The general manifestations are observed only at the time of seroconversion. Modifications of the CSF content are similar to those observed in classical GBS.

Subacute multifocal neuropathy

This is the most original pattern of neuropathy observed in HIV patients, before the onset of cellular immunodepression. A sensory or sensorimotor deficit often predominates in the lower limbs. Paraesthesias and spontaneous pains are common. They are bilateral but often predominate on one side, or can affect the territory of a nerve trunk or of a spinal root. They often progress over a few weeks, and affect the upper limbs. The CSF usually shows an increase in protein content and mild pleocytosis with normal glucose levels. The outcome of these neuropathies is usually good. Patients improve spontaneously or after treatment with corticosteroids.

In nerve biopsies of patients with subacute multifocal neuropathy, mixed axonal and demyelinative lesions of nerve fibres are associated with mild inflammatory infiltrates. In most cases, perivascular cuffing is associated with endoneurial inflammatory infiltrates, mainly made up of CD8+ T-lymphocytes and macrophages. In a few patients we found necrotising arteritis of the type observed in polyarteritis nodosa, both in nerve and in muscle specimens.

Distal symmetrical axonal polyneuropathy

Distal symmetrical neuropathies originally represent the most common type of peripheral neuropathy in HIV patients, especially at the late stage of the HIV infection. Both feet are affected simultaneously by painful sensations, often of the burning type, associated with painful contact dysaesthesias which render examination difficult. Painful retraction of the calf muscles occurs. Motor involvement is usually absent or moderate. Slight pyramidal tract involvement is common. The ankle reflexes are absent or decreased; the other tendon reflexes are often brisk.

Cytomegalovirus (CMV) neuropathy

CMV neuropathy is a treatable neuropathy that occurs at the late stage of immunodepression [24]. CMV infection represents the most common viral opportunistic infection in AIDS, affecting 15-35% of AIDS patients. Its most common clinical manifestation is retinitis, with vision loss, that is often bilateral. The diagnosis of CMV neuropathy should not be missed since it is accessible to specific treatment by ganciclovir or foscarnet. In most cases, patients with proven CMV neuropathy have AIDS with opportunistic infections, profound immunodepression, fever, cachexia, a CD4+ T-cell count below 50 per ml, and CMV retinitis, but in some patients, CMV neuropathy is the first and only opportunistic infection and occurs in patients in a relatively good general condition.

The different patterns of CMV neuropathy include:

- the polyradiculoneuropathic pattern in which patients develop, within a few days or weeks, a sensorimotor deficit of the lower spinal roots, or a complete cauda equina syndrome, with sphincter disturbances;
- the multifocal pattern with lesions of spinal roots, nerve trunks, and sometimes cranial nerve involvement;
- severe CNS manifestations including necrotic myelitis and encephalitis;
- CSF abnormalities that can be observed in this setting such as a high protein content (more than 10g/L in one of our patients), pleocytosis with a polymorphonuclear leucocyte reaction and a decrease in CSF glucose. The CSF can, however, remain normal.

The multifocal, necrotic, endoneurial lesions with a neutrophilic cell response, which may look like multiple endoneurial microabcesses, seem unique to this viral agent. These lesions markedly differ from those observed in other types of HIV-associated neuropathies (Figure 5). Specific lesions of the CNS, with predominant infection of glial and endothelial cells, are often found on postmortem examination. Although infrequent, distinct neurological syndromes caused by CMV continue to cause high mortality among AIDS patients. Survival depends upon the use of effective antiviral therapy against CMV and the early introduction of HAART.

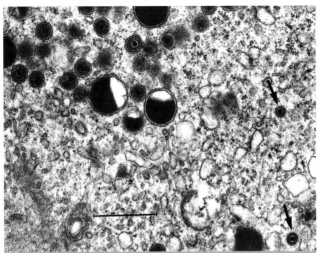

Figure 5. Electron micrograph of a nerve biopsy specimen from a patient with AIDS and multifocal neuropathy due to opportunistic infection with cytomegalovirus. The arrows point to CMV virions present in an endoneurial cell. (Uranyl acetate and lead citrate staining. Bar: 1μm.)

Malignant lymphomas

Malignant lymphomas, which may complicate the immunosuppression of AIDS can induce focal or multifocal nerve lesions by invading spinal roots or nerve trunks.

Toxic neuropathy in AIDS

The antiviral drug 2',3'-dideoxyinosine (DDI), an antagonist of DNA viral synthesis, induces a distal symmetrical sensory polyneuropathy in 7% of patients receiving less than 12mg/kg/day. The symptoms disappear after withdrawal of the drug, which can be started again later at lower doses. Others have found neuropathy in 2% of patients only.

➲ Key points

- The neuropathy induced by *Mycobacterium leprae* mainly depends on the immunological response of the host.

- In lepromatous leprous neuropathy, nerves contain many bacilli, while in the tuberculoid form bacilli are scarce.

- Reversal reactions that occur during treatment can destroy peripheral nerves more than the infection itself.

- Lyme disease is a meningoradiculoneuritis due to infection with *Borrelia burgdorferi* which is transmitted via a tick bite.

- Lyme disease is a self-limiting disease which may, however, leave residual deficits.

- HIV infection can be associated with a variety of peripheral neuropathies.

References

1.   Ridley DS. Histological classification and the immunological spectrum of leprosy. *Bull WHO* 1974; 51: 451-65.

2.   Bloom BR, Godal T. Selective primary health care: strategies for control of disease in the developing world. V. Leprosy. *Reviews of Infect Diseases* 1983; 5: 765-80.

3.   Hansen GA. Under sgeiser angaende spedalskhedensarasger tiedels uf forte sammem med forstander Hartwig. *Norske Mag Laegevidensj* 1874; 4: S1.

4.   WHO. Progress in Leprosy Control, Indonesia 1991-2008. *Weekly Epidemiological Record* 2010; 85: 249-62.

5.   Tzourio C, Said G, Milan J. Asymptomatic nerve hypertrophy in lepromatous leprosy: a clinical, electrophysiological and morphological study. *J Neurol* 1992; 239: 367-74.

6.   de Freitas MR, Said G. Leprous neuropathy. *Handb Clin Neurol* 2013; 115: 499-514.

7.   Ridley DS, Jopling WH. Classification of leprosy according to immunity. A five-group system. *Int J Lepr Other Mycobact Dis* 1966; 34: 255-73.

8.   Lockwood DN, Sarno E, Smith WC. Classification of leprosy patients: searching for the perfect solution? *Lepr Rev* 2007; 78: 317-20.

9.   Modlin RL. The innate immune response in leprosy. *Curr Opin Immunol* 2010; 22: 48-54.

10. Job CK. Recent histopathological studies in leprosy, with particular reference to early diagnosis and leprous neuropathy. *Int J Lepr* 2007; 79: 75-83.

11. Lipschütz B. Weiterer Beitrag zur Kenntis des "Erythema chronicum migrans". *Arch Dermatlo Syph* 1923; 143: 365-74.

12. Garin C, Bujadoux C. Paralysie par les tiques. *J Med Lyon* 1922; 3: 765-7.

13. Bannwarth A. Zur Klinik und Pathogenese der "chronischen lymphocytaren Meningitis". *Arch Psychiatr Nervenkr* 1944; 117: 161-85.

14. Steere AC, Malawista SE, Snydman DR, *et al*. Lyme arthritis: an epidemic of oligoarticular arthritis in children and adults in three Connecticut communities. *Arthritis Rheum* 1977; 20: 7-17.

15. Hansen K, Crone C, Kristoferitsch W. Lyme neuroborreliosis. *Handb Clin Neurol* 2013; 115: 559-75.

16. Steere AC. Lyme disease. *N Engl J Med* 1989; 321: 586-96.

17. Pachner AR, Steere AC. The triad of neurologic manifestations of Lyme disease: meningitis, cranial neuritis, and radiculoneuritis. *Neurology* 1985; 35: 47-53.

18. Steere AC, Batsford WP, Weinberg M, *et al*. Lyme carditis: cardiac abnormalities of Lyme disease. *Ann Intern Med* 1980; 93: 8-16.

19. Kruger H, Reuss K, Pulz M, *et al*. Meningoradiculitis and encephalomyelitis due to *Borrelia burgdorferi*: a follow-up study of 72 patients over 27 years. *J Neurol* 1989; 236: 322-8.

20. Steere AC, Hutchinson GJ, Rahn DW, *et al*. Treatment of early manifestations of Lyme disease. *Ann Intern Med* 1983; 99: 22-6.

21. Snider WD, Simpson DM, Nielsen S, *et al*. Neurological complications of acquired immune deficiency syndrome: analysis of 50 patients. *Ann Neurol* 1983; 14: 403-18.

22. Lipkin WI, Parry G, Kiprov DD, Abrams D. Inflammatory neuropathy in homosexual men with lymphadenopathy. *Neurology* 1985; 35: 1479-83.

23. Gabbai AA, Castelo A, Oliveira AS. HIV peripheral neuropathy. *Handb Clin Neurol* 2013; 115: 515-29.

24. Said G, Lacroix C, Chemouilli P, *et al*. Cytomegalovirus (CMV) neuropathy in AIDS: a clinical and pathological study. *Ann Neurol* 1991; 29: 139-46.

Chapter 8

Diabetic and uraemic neuropathies

Overview

In this chapter the complications of diabetes on the peripheral nervous system are discussed, in particular, axonal sensory neuropathy, as well as the less common manifestations of diabetes. In this review we will also consider the classical aspects of diabetic neuropathy, the recent contributions on the subject, the current treatments of diabetic neuropathy and the practical management of diabetic patients with neuropathy. In addition, the effects of severe renal impairment on the peripheral nervous system are described.

Diabetic neuropathies

Introduction

Diabetes mellitus is the commonest cause of neuropathy in industrialised countries. It can present with a variety of manifestations including distal symmetrical polyneuropathy, autonomic, at times life-threatening autonomic dysfunction, and focal or multifocal involvement of the peripheral nervous system. In addition to these classic aspects, some inflammatory neuropathies, such as chronic inflammatory demyelinating polyneuropathy (CIDP), seem more common in diabetic patients who are exposed, just as non-diabetic subjects, to all the other causes of neuropathy.

Epidemiology

In 2013, according to the International Diabetes Federation, an estimated 381 million people have diabetes [1]. Its incidence is increasing rapidly and by 2030, this number is estimated to almost double. Thus, 8.3% of adults are estimated to have diabetes and 316 million people have an impaired glucose tolerance test. The largest increases will take place in the regions where developing economies are predominant.

The prevalence of neuropathy in several population-based surveys is around 30% in studies using restrictive definitions [2]. The prevalence of sensory symptoms or signs that included numbness, a loss of feeling, pain or tingling, a decreased ability to feel hot or cold, was found to be 30.2% among patients with type 1 diabetes [3]. The prevalence of diabetic peripheral neuropathy increases with age and with the duration of diabetes until it is present in more than 50% of type 1 diabetics aged over 60 years [4]. It is important to take into account that the onset of type 2 diabetes is estimated to occur 4-7 years before clinical diagnosis [3]. Furthermore, at least 30% of people in the US with type 2 diabetes are undiagnosed.

To summarise the findings of the various epidemiological studies:

- diabetic neuropathy may complicate type 1 or type 2 diabetes;
- neuropathy may be present at the time of discovery of type 2 diabetes due to the presence of undiscovered diabetes during the preceding years or decades;
- the prevalence of neuropathy increases with duration and poor diabetic control.

Clinicopathological aspects

Since diabetic neuropathy was first described, the diversity of clinical manifestations has led to several classification systems. Although no satisfactory classification can account for the variety of manifestations of diabetic neuropathy, most of them fall into:

- the distal symmetrical sensorimotor, length-dependent, polyneuropathy;
- autonomic neuropathy;
- focal and multifocal neuropathy.

Distal symmetrical diabetic polyneuropathy

Distal symmetrical polyneuropathy is by far the most common neuropathic pattern in diabetes. It is a predominantly sensory neuropathy with no motor deficit in most cases. Distal motor deficit, if present, is usually slight and occurs mainly in the most severe forms.

Distal symmetrical predominantly sensory polyneuropathy

Distal symmetrical sensory polyneuropathy (DSSP) has an insidious onset and is the most common pattern of neuropathy in diabetic patients. It usually becomes symptomatic several years after the onset of type 1 diabetes but often is the initial presentation of type 2 diabetes (mature onset). Inaugural positive manifestations of sensory neuropathy include numbness, burning feet, a pins and needles sensation, and lancinating pains which are often worse at night. The sensory neuropathy can be totally asymptomatic and detected only by systematic neurological examination of the feet. In such cases the neuropathy is identified following painless trauma or burns, or by trophic changes with plantar ulcers or neuro-osteoarthropathy (Charcot's joint).

Dependent on the degree of damage to the peripheral nerves, the distal symmetrical sensory loss can be restricted to the toes, extend over the feet, spread over the legs or higher above the knee level. When sensory loss extends above the knee, there is likely to be the development of sensory signs and symptoms in the fingers with spread up over the hands and the forearms as it progresses proximally. Subsequently, the anterior aspect of the trunk can become affected due to the involvement of the distal territory of the sensory nerve fibres of the intercostal nerves. In the most severe cases the top of the scalp can be affected due to the involvement of the longest fibres of the trigeminal nerve and, exceptionally, loss of sensation can spread over the whole body. This pattern of distribution of sensory loss suggests a fibre-length degeneration of nerve fibres. Sensory loss predominates, but this is not restricted to thermal and pain perception.

The maximum dissociation of function between small and large fibres occurs in the so-called 'pseudosyringomyelic type' which was originally reported by Vergely (1893) in diabetic patients [5]. In small fibre diabetic DSSP, the length-related sensory loss mainly affects pain and temperature perception and leads to the occurrence of painless burns, persistent foot ulcers and neuropathic osteoarthropathy (Charcot's joint) [6]. The loss of large myelinated fibres can lead to a disturbance of light touch sense, to a sensibility to pressure, vibration and joint position sense, in addition to that of other proprioceptive afferent fibres. This can result in an increased instability of posture with, in the most severe cases, a positive Romberg's sign. Although this 'pseudotabetic' pattern of diabetic neuropathy was recognised more than a century ago by Charcot in 1890, it seems rather uncommon nowadays [7].

Painful symmetrical polyneuropathy

Acute painful neuropathy and cachexia occur in newly diagnosed diabetic patients [8]. Sensory loss is mild or absent and reflex loss or depression are not invariable [9]. These severe manifestations usually subside within 10 months, and improve with good diabetic control. Paradoxically, precipitation of an acute painful neuropathy has been observed after the establishment of tight glycaemic control following a long period of extremely poor diabetic control [10].

Motor involvement in distal symmetrical diabetic neuropathy

Mild distal muscle weakness and wasting may accompany severe DSSP, but predominantly a motor neuropathy is not a feature of distal neuropathy in diabetic patients. Motor deficit is a late event in the natural history of DSSP. When observed in this setting, motor deficit is always bilateral, distal and roughly symmetrical. Its onset is also more gradual and indolent, but with an unrelenting course. The occurrence of a predominantly motor distal involvement in diabetic patients is more suggestive of a superimposed motor neuron disease or of an inflammatory polyneuropathy.

Trophic changes in distal symmetrical sensory polyneuropathy

Trophic changes observed in diabetic patients include foot ulceration and neurogenic osteoarthropathy (Charcot's joint). These complications, which result from loss of pain sensation, also occur in a number of conditions that associate loss of pain sensation with preservation of normal or subnormal strength, leading to painless trauma and the development of plantar ulcers and osteoarthropathy.

Foot ulceration

Foot lesions are common in middle-aged and elderly diabetics. Peripheral neuropathy causes sensory impairment and weakness of the intrinsic foot muscles, leading to foot deformities in advanced forms. The earliest change is often a callus, which may recur despite regular foot care. In other cases, the first manifestation is a painless phlyctenular lesion of the plantar aspect of the foot. In both cases, they are painless and are associated with a loss of pain sensation over the feet. Chronic ulcers most commonly arise on the sole of the foot, in the region of the metatarsal heads. In addition to the sensory loss, the micro- and macro-ischaemic effects of diabetes contributes to foot ulceration.

Neuropathic osteoarthropathy

Painless foot deformity, sometimes of acute onset, is a major sign of this complication. On X-ray, feet may show increased radiotransparency, painless fractures especially affecting the metatarsal bone, disruption of articular surfaces, and disorganisation of joints, especially of the metatarsophalangeal joints. Penetration of bacteria through neuropathic ulcers can lead to chronic osteomyelitis, and to the overestimation of the extent of irreversible bone destruction of neuropathic origin. Neuro-osteoarthropathy (Charcot's joint) has an incidence of approximately 2% per annum in patients with diabetic peripheral neuropathy [11].

Autonomic neuropathy in diabetic patients

In 1945, Rundles identified most manifestations of diabetic dysautonomia [12]. Clinical cardiovascular disturbances usually start with a reduction or loss of R-R variations during standing or breathing. After some time, months, usually, there is a resting tachycardia, then the heart rate may return to normal values but without normal variations. Postural hypotension (a fall in systolic blood pressure of more than 30mmHg on changing from a lying to a standing position, without increasing the heart rate) may be an extremely disabling symptom of autonomic neuropathy with postural syncope. Postural hypotension can be aggravated by tricyclic antidepressants which are often used for the treatment of chronic pain in diabetic neuropathy. A review of concomitant medication, including medication such as diuretics that may be compounding postural hypotension with hypovolaemia, should be undertaken prior to starting treatments such as fludrocortisone.

Gastroparesis is a common manifestation of disturbances of alimentary tract function. It is often asymptomatic, but at times may be revealed by a sensation of fullness. Less commonly it is accompanied by vomiting. Gastroparesis may result in poor diabetic control with hypoglycaemia because of the stagnation of food in the stomach. Diabetic diarrhoea occurs at night or after meals and is watery. It may be accompanied by faecal incontinence due to reduced pressure in the internal anal sphincter.

Bladder atony leads to the presence of a large residual volume after micturition, sometimes complicated by infection. Retrograde ejaculation is frequent in patients with an atonic bladder. Impotence which can be evaluated by continuous nocturnal penile tumescence and rigidity monitoring, is a common complication in male diabetic patients. Vascular and psychogenic factors as well as ageing may also contribute to impotence.

Unawareness of hypoglycaemia may complicate autonomic neuropathy due to failure of catecholamine release, which induces cutaneous vasoconstriction and sweating. The release of pancreatic glucagon in response to hypoglycaemia, which is mediated by the vagus, may also be deficient in diabetic autonomic neuropathy and lead to a more rapid onset of hypoglycaemia.

Disorders of sweating are common in the feet. Heat intolerance and profuse sweating over the head and upper trunk may be due to anhydrosis over the legs, lower trunk and sometimes the arms with compensatory sweating elsewhere. Abnormal pupillary responses are common in diabetic patients. The two most striking signs are miosis and reduced light reflexes, the measurement of which can provide useful autonomic function tests.

Pathological aspects of distal symmetrical diabetic neuropathy

Abnormalities reported in diabetic neuropathy include fibres undergoing axonal degeneration, primary demyelination which results from Schwann cell dysfunction, and secondary segmental demyelination, which is related to impairment of the axonal control of myelination. Remyelination, proliferation of Schwann cells, atrophy of denervated bands of Schwann cells, onion bulb formation and hypertrophy of the basal lamina may also be observed (Figures 1-3). Dying-back fibres and fibres with distal sprouting of the proximal stump,

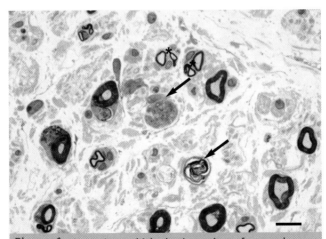

Figure 1. One-micron-thick plastic section of a sural nerve biopsy of a patient with a severe sensory and autonomic diabetic polyneuropathy. Several fibres are undergoing axonal degeneration (arrows), while a few clusters of regenerating axons can be seen (asterisks). (Bar 10μm.)

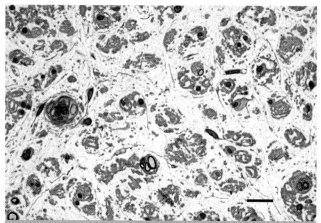

Figure 2. One-micron-thick plastic section of a sural nerve biopsy of a patient with an extremely severe sensory and autonomic diabetic polyneuropathy. Note the almost complete disappearance of nerve fibres. (Thionine blue staining. Bar 10µm.)

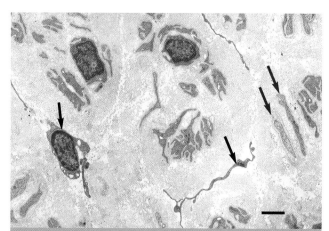

Figure 3. Electron micrograph of a sural nerve biopsy of a patient with poorly controlled type 1 diabetes and longstanding sensory polyneuropathy. No nerve fibre, myelinated or unmyelinated, can be seen on this field; only fibroblasts (black arrows) and Schwann cell processes (red arrows) can be identified. This is the most severe pathological aspect of length-dependent diabetic neuropathy. (Uranyl acetate and lead citrate staining. Bar 1µm.)

subsequent to degeneration of the distal axon, have also been identified in length-dependent diabetic neuropathy [6].

Focal and multifocal neuropathy

A number of focal and, occasionally, multifocal neuropathic syndromes occur in the setting of diabetes mellitus. They include cranial nerve involvement, limb and truncal neuropathies, and proximal diabetic neuropathy (PDN) of the lower limbs. In this group of neuropathies the disorder tends to occur both in men and women over the age of 50, most with longstanding type 1 or type 2 diabetes. It is relatively common to see patients with this pattern of neuropathy with no history of diabetes. The severity of diabetes is often mild. In this population focal neuropathy often coexists with silent or pauci-symptomatic DSSP. The long-term prognosis of focal neuropathy is good in most cases but sequelae occur in some patients with proximal diabetic neuropathy.

Cranial diabetic neuropathy
Oculomotor nerve palsies are the most common if not the only cranial neuropathy observed in diabetic patients.

It is interesting to note that the frequency of oculomotor palsy in diabetic patients is between 1-2%. The sixth and third cranial nerves are the most commonly affected. In virtually all cases diabetic ophthalmoplegia occurs in diabetic patients over 50 years of age. The onset is rapid, within a day or two. In many cases the patient experiences pain ranging from a few hours to a few days before noticing diplopia. Pain is usually aching, behind or above the eye, and sometimes more diffuse but always on the same side as the oculomotor palsy. Pain does not persist after the onset of diplopia.

Oculomotor dysfunction is often incomplete when the third nerve is involved. One or two muscles only may be paralysed. Ptosis is marked, the eye is deviated outward when the internal rectus muscle is affected and the patient is unable to move the eye medially, upward or downward. Pupillary innervation is spared in most cases. Spontaneous and complete recovery invariably occurs within 2-3 months, independently of the quality of control of hyperglycaemia.

Focal limb neuropathy

Isolated involvement of peripheral nerves of the limbs, including radial, median and ulnar nerves in the upper limbs and of the peroneal nerve for the lower limbs, seldom occurs in diabetic patients. Whilst we have seen occasional examples of isolated involvement of the radial, median and ulnar nerves, such cases are extremely rare and should always be investigated as in non-diabetic patients. Proximal weakness of the upper limbs, as it appears in the lower limbs, is very uncommon. In the lower limbs, the most common pattern of focal neuropathy is characterised by proximal sensory and motor manifestations.

Proximal diabetic neuropathy of the lower limbs

Diabetic patients, usually over the age of 50, may also present proximal neuropathy of the lower limbs characterised by a variable degree of pain and sensory loss associated with uni- or bilateral proximal muscle weakness and atrophy. This syndrome, which was originally described by Bruns in 1890 [13], has been subsequently reported under the terms of proximal diabetic neuropathy (PDN) [14, 15] or femoral-sciatic neuropathy. The mean age at diagnosis was 62 years. Men were more often affected than females.

The onset of the neuropathy is acute or subacute. The patient complains of numbness or pain of the anterior aspect of the thigh, often of the burning type and worse at night. Difficulty in walking and climbing stairs occurs, due to weakness of the quadriceps and iliopsoas muscles. Muscle wasting is also an early and common phenomenon, which is often easier to palpate than to see in fatter patients (Figure 4). The patellar reflex is decreased or more often abolished. The syndrome progresses over weeks or months in most cases, then stabilises, and spontaneous pains decrease, sometimes rapidly. In many instances, as in those originally reported, there is no marked or any sensory loss, as emphasized by Garland [16]. In approximately one third of patients there is a definite sensory loss over the anterior aspect of the thigh, and in others a painful contact dysaesthesia in the distribution of the cutaneous branches of the femoral nerve, without a definite sensory loss.

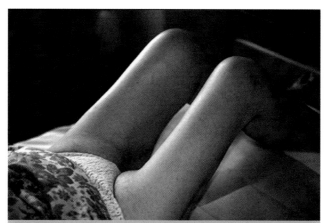

Figure 4. Massive amyotrophy of the right thigh in a patient with type 2 diabetes and severe proximal neuropathy of the lower limbs.

In most cases the patient's condition improves after months, but sequelae, including disabling weakness and amyotrophy, sensory loss and patellar areflexia, are common. In a survey of long-term follow-up of up to 14 years, recovery began after a median interval of 3 months (range 1-12 months)[17]. Pain was the first symptom to improve, resolution being comparatively rapid, beginning within a few weeks and being almost complete by 12 months. Residual discomfort in the patients of Coppack and Watkins took up to 3 years to subside. Motor recovery was satisfactory but seven patients complained of some persisting weakness. Significant wasting of the thigh was evident in half of the cases [17]. Relapses, on the other hand, are common, sometimes in spite of good diabetic control. In one fifth of patients that we investigated for this syndrome, relapses occurred within a few months, the same proportion as in the Coppack and Watkins study. Thus, the clinical features of PDN with its frequent motor involvement, asymmetrical deficit, gradual yet often incomplete spontaneous recovery, markedly differ from those of DSSP in which the length-dependent symmetrical sensory deficit is associated with motor signs only in extreme cases, and virtually never improves spontaneously. In the syndrome described by Garland as 'diabetic amyotrophy', motor manifestations are more prominent but lesions of the sensory branch of the femoral nerve are also present in such patients [18]. Some authors have advocated the use of steroids in the acute phase, but this is based on case reports rather than trial evidence [19].

Pathological aspects of PDN

Study of biopsy specimens of the intermediate cutaneous nerve of the thigh, a sensory branch of the femoral nerve which conveys sensation from the anterior aspect of the thigh, a territory commonly involved in PDN, showed lesions characteristic of severe nerve ischaemia in a large proportion of patients [18, 20]. Recent occlusion of perineurial blood vessels and perivascular, perineurial and subperineurial inflammatory infiltration with mononuclear cells were demonstrated in some, along with axonal degeneration of the majority of nerve fibres (Figure 5). In other patients, lesions of nerve fibres and of endoneurial capillaries were similar to those observed in the sural nerve in diabetic patients with symptomatic DSSP.

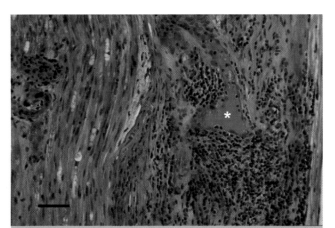

Figure 5. Section of a biopsy specimen of the superficial peroneal nerve from a patient with multifocal neuropathy affecting the femoral nerve and the peroneal nerves on both sides. Note the important inflammatory infiltrate made up of mononuclear cells surrounding the venule (asterisk). (Hematein eosin staining. Bar 20μm.)

The presence of inflammatory infiltrates does not preclude spontaneous recovery.

Thoracic neuropathy

Truncal or thoracoabdominal neuropathy occurs almost only in older diabetic subjects [21]. It is unilateral or predominantly so. The onset is abrupt or rapid, with pain or dysaesthesia as the main features. The pain may have a radicular distribution and is made worse by contact and at night. Weakness of abdominal muscles can occur.

Multifocal diabetic neuropathy

In a small proportion of diabetic patients, a multifocal neuropathy is observed with successive or simultaneous involvement, over months, of roots and nerves of the lower limbs, the trunk and the upper extremities. In our series of 22 patients, three patients had a relapsing course. A painful multifocal sensory-motor deficit had progressed over 2-12 months. The distal lower limbs were involved in all patients, unilaterally in seven, bilaterally in others, with an asynchronous onset in most cases. In addition, a proximal deficit of the lower limbs was present on one side in seven patients, on both sides in six. Thoracic radiculoneuropathy was present bilaterally in two patients, unilaterally in one. The ulnar nerve was involved in one patient, the radial nerve in two. The cerebrospinal fluid (CSF) protein ranged from 0.40-3.55g/L, with a mean of 0.87g/L. Electrophysiological testing showed severe, multifocal, axonal nerve lesions in all cases [22]. Necrotising vasculitis of perineurial and endoneurial blood vessels was found in six patients, endoneurial seepage of red cells in 11 specimens, endoneurial haemorrhage in five, and post-haemorrhagic ferric iron deposits in 10 patients. Besides the high frequency both of endoneurial bleeding and of inflammatory infiltrates, occlusion of small and middle-sized epineurial and perineurial arteries differentiates multifocal diabetic neuropathy (MDN) from DSSP. The outcome is better in MDN than in DSSP. Improvement occurs in all patients after a few months, but long-term sequelae are common.

Non-diabetic neuropathies more common in diabetic patients

In addition to specific neuropathies, diabetic patients seem more prone to develop some types of neuropathy than non-diabetic patients (a double hit).

Increased liability to pressure palsy

Pressure palsy is more common in diabetic individuals. Carpal tunnel syndrome occurs in 12% of diabetic patients, and the incidence of ulnar neuropathy due to microlesions at the elbow level is high in diabetic patients too.

Acquired inflammatory demyelinative polyneuropathy

Inflammatory, predominantly demyelinating neuropathy also must be differentiated from diabetic polyneuropathy, and may occur with a greater frequency in this population. This diagnosis must be suspected when an acute or subacute, often predominantly motor, demyelinative polyneuropathy occurs in a diabetic patient. Electrophysiological features are those of a demyelinative neuropathy [23, 24]. The course and response to treatment is often the same as in non-diabetic patients.

Mucormycosis

This rare condition is an acute disease that successively affects the air cavities of the face, the orbit and the brain, as a result of proliferation of a fungus of the class *Phycomyceta*. In 36% of cases it is associated with diabetes, especially diabetic acidosis. This may present with an episode of rhinological involvement with epistaxis, violent headaches, and orbitonasal pain with swelling of the lids and ophthalmoplegia. The disease spreads to the meninges and to the brain through the arteries, inducing thrombosis of the ophthalmic then of the internal carotid artery, with subsequent hemiplegia. The prognosis is extremely poor. The diagnosis should be made as soon as possible with a biopsy of the nasal lesions which allows identification of the causative phycomycete and the start of treatment.

Renal failure in diabetic patients

Diabetes is the leading cause of end-stage renal disease in the US and Europe. Renal insufficiency is a common complication of diabetic nephropathy, which can necessitate periodic dialysis and/or a renal transplant. In this population with both diabetes and major renal failure, neuropathy is common and often severe. The deleterious effect of renal failure on nerve function is responsible for much of the severe motor deficit, sometimes of rapid onset, that patients may present in this context. Recovery from motor deficit is usually good after kidney transplantation.

Differential diagnosis

In focal neuropathy occurring in diabetic patients, a neuropathy of another origin must always be excluded. In patients with ophthalmoplegia, the preservation of pupillary motricity in a nearly complete third cranial nerve palsy strongly suggests a diabetic origin; however, even in such cases, it is wise to perform non-invasive investigations of the area. Magnetic resonance angiography will rule out the possibility of a compressive lesion of the third cranial nerve by a large aneurysm of the carotid artery within the cavernous sinus, an aneurysm in the posterior communicating artery, or a fusiform aneurysm at the top of the basilar artery. Imaging will also help to exclude tumours occurring at the base of the brain or in the basal skull. In patients with progressive involvement of several cranial nerves without imaging abnormalities, examination of the CSF may detect malignant cells characteristic of a carcinomatous meningitis. In diabetic patients who develop a focal or multifocal neuropathy of the limbs, other causes than diabetes should also be considered. The first step in this context is to determine if the lesions are located in the spinal roots or in the peripheral nerves, a distinction which may be difficult clinically and electrophysiologically. In addition, the lesions may be mixed. A nerve and a muscle biopsy should be performed, especially in focal or multifocal neuropathy. When a diabetic patient develops proximal weakness without much pain, a superimposed cause of motor neuropathy or of motor neuron disease must be considered, and appropriate investigations undertaken.

Nerve conduction studies

A number of electrophysiological studies have been performed in diabetic patients. Changes in conduction velocity can be detected in asymptomatic patients but their presence is not predictive of the occurrence of symptomatic neuropathy. Systematic electrophysiological evaluation of diabetic patients does not seem advisable. In symptomatic diabetic neuropathy there is a mixture of a slowing of nerve conduction velocity due to demyelination and a loss of large myelinated fibres, and a decrease in nerve action potentials also due to loss of axons, and increased temporal dispersion. A purely demyelinative neuropathy is exceptional in diabetic patients and is more suggestive, for instance, of the occurrence of a demyelinating neuropathy of inflammatory or dysglobulinaemic origin. Systematic electrophysiological testing of diabetic patients with typical peripheral neuropathy is not necessary.

Pathophysiology of diabetic neuropathy

Both metabolic and ischaemic mechanisms may play a role in diabetic neuropathies: the metabolic factor seems to prevail in DSSN and in mild forms of PDN, while a superimposed inflammatory process and ischaemic nerve lesions seem responsible for severe forms of PDN. The thickening and hyalinisation of the walls of small blood vessels suggests a role for nerve ischaemia in diabetic neuropathy.

The role of the accumulation of polyols observed in animals also occurs in humans but whether this accumulation in nerves leads to neuropathy is not established. The usefulness of treatment with aldose-reductase inhibitors has not been confirmed. The reduction of protein synthesis and transport has been found in animal models and may account for the occurrence of dying-back fibres in the nerves. Impairment of axonal elongation and calibre growth of regenerating fibres has been found in diabetic rats, along with downregulation of mRNA and neurofilament protein expression. A number of other factors and mechanisms may play a role [25, 26].

Treatment of diabetic neuropathy (➲ see case studies on pp118-22)

Preventative treatment
Prevention of diabetic neuropathy and of its complications remains the best treatment. Optimum diabetic control diminishes the risk of developing a disabling peripheral neuropathy, but it is not often achievable, because it carries a higher risk of hypoglycaemia. Prevention of the consequences of hyperglycaemia on nerves can include the use of aldose-reductase

inhibitors, where the efficacy of such treatment has been demonstrated. Most aldose-reductase inhibitors have actually failed to significantly improve patients with diabetic neuropathy.

The prevention of complications of diabetic neuropathy includes prevention of trophic changes in the feet. Diabetics need advice about foot care and footwear and about the protection of hyposensitive areas and pressure points, to prevent the occurrence of painless ulcers and decrease the risk of bone infection. Prevention and treatment of the diabetic foot are best given in specialised foot clinics. Diabetics with sensory loss also need advice about painless burns and injuries.

Treatment of symptoms

In focal neuropathy, including cranial nerve palsy, proximal diabetic neuropathy or truncal neuropathy, the course is self-limiting with a good spontaneous recovery, in most cases within a few months. Yet control of pain may be difficult in these neuropathies as well as in symmetrical neuropathies. Carbamazepine, diphenylhydantoin, gabapentin, pregabalin, duloxetine or clonazepam are sometimes useful or paracetamol associated with codeine. Tricyclic antidepressants (imipramine, amitryptyline, etc.) are often effective. The usual dose varies from 30-150mg per day. Tricyclic antidepressants may aggravate postural hypotension. Only symptomatic postural hypotension requires treatment. The most effective treatment is 9-fluorohydrocortisone which carries a risk of hypertension in a lying position.

Distal symmetrical sensorimotor length-dependent polyneuropathy

There is no specific treatment for distal symmetrical polyneuropathy. Only the complications of this condition can be treated or prevented, including trophic changes, neuropathic pain (see Chapter 11 – Neuropathic pain – for more detail) and the symptoms of autonomic neuropathy.

Autonomic neuropathy

Treatment of autonomic neuropathy relates mostly to treating symptomatic postural hypotension. Metoclopramide and domperidone can be helpful in patients with diabetic gastroparesis. Diarrhoea can be controlled by Imodium® or by octreotide, a somatostatin analogue. Viagra and tadalafil can be tried in patients complaining of sexual impotence.

Sensory ataxia and diabetic neuropathy

Richard, a 66-year-old man, had a 35-year history of non-insulin-dependent diabetes complicated by background retinopathy, micro- and macroangiopathy, hypothyroidism, and mild renal insufficiency. He was on permanent anticoagulation for atrial fibrillation.

In August 2011, he started to complain of numbness in both feet, and quickly felt balance problems. Two months later, the numbness had progressed to the hands.

Electromyography (EMG) was performed in October 2011 which failed to detect any sensory action potential in the lower limbs and in the median and radial nerves on both sides. F-wave distal latency of the right posterior tibial nerve was increased.

The patient was referred to the Neurology Department of the hospital in November 2011. His strength was normal in all four limbs. He had a fibre-length-dependent alteration of superficial sensation predominantly on pinprick and temperature sensation. All four limbs and the anterior trunk were affected. Position sense was impaired in the right foot. He had sensory ataxia. All tendon reflexes were abolished. There was no meaningful autonomic disturbance. The CSF contained 1g/L protein and there were no cells found (0 cell/ml in the CSF = normal).

The superficial peroneal nerve was biopsied under local anaesthesia. The density of nerve fibres was reduced to 40% of normal values. There were many clusters of regenerating fibres and most surviving fibres were hypomyelinated. There were no inflammatory infiltrates. The endoneurial blood vessels showed features of diabetic microangiopathy.

Continued overleaf

Sensory ataxia and diabetic neuropathy *continued*

A large majority of the isolated teased fibres showed segmental abnormalities with demyelinating-remyelinating features and short internodes. A few fibres were at a late stage of Wallerian degeneration.

Ultra-thin sections of the nerve specimens stained with uranyl acetate and lead citrate were examined under the electron microscope. The only salient feature was the striking reduction of the density of unmyelinated axons, in agreement with a longstanding diabetic polyneuropathy. An isolated endoneurial capillary showed changes suggestive of diabetic microaneurysms.

In November 2011 there was a marked increase of sensory deficit with minimal weakness in the hands (strength 4/5). The diagnosis of chronic inflammatory demyelinated polyneuropathy (CIDP) was considered and treatment with high-dose intravenous immunoglobulins (IVIGs) was given from November 13 to November 16, without success.

In December the patient was quadriplegic. Methylprednisolone was then given intravenously (500mg/d for 5 days), followed by oral prednisone (65mg/day). The patient started to improve after a week. After 2 months on corticosteroids the Norris score was 36/81. In March 2012, the Norris score was 78/81 (prednisone was gradually decreased from 65mg to 40mg/d). Corticosteroids were tapered over a few months. The patient remained well neurologically, until his death which occurred 2 years later, from ischaemic heart disease.

This patient had a CIDP which complicated the course of a mild diabetic polyneuropathy. It is worth noting the good response of CIDP to corticosteroids after the failure of IVIGs.

Severe length-dependent diabetic polyneuropathy

Rachel, a 24-year-old, had been diagnosed with type 1 diabetes since the age of 8 years and had been treated with insulin ever since, with poor glycaemic control. Her glycated haemoglobin (HbA1c) was often above 10%. She had micro- and macroproteinuria for years. She was referred at age 24.

Previously, at age 22, she started to notice that she could not feel the temperature of the water in her bath but light touch remained normal. In the following years she experienced increasing postural hypotension, with dizziness and fainting upon standing. Her blood pressure which was 140/65mmHg in the lying position fell to 60mmHg systolic pressure within less than a minute upon standing (diastolic pressure was extremely low), with dizziness and fainting if she did not lie down quickly. Her pulse rate was 76 per minute when lying down but remained unchanged upon standing, which is characteristic of neurogenic postural hypotension. In addition to life-threatening postural hypotension she had episodes of vomiting and gastroparesis which increased hypotension. Postural hypotension responded well to treatment with 9-alpha-fluorohydrocortisone, 100μg/day.

She gradually developed proliferative retinopathy and nephropathy with subsequent renal failure. At the age of 32 years, she had lost temperature sense over the whole of her body, but light touch and vibratory sensation had not changed. Muscle strength and position sense remained normal.

Periodic haemodialysis was started when she was 33 years old; she died a year later from septic shock.

This case illustrates the occurrence of extremely severe small fibre neuropathy affecting temperature and pain sensation, with life-threatening autonomic disturbances.

Late-onset sensory diabetic polyneuropathy

Jack is a 52-year-old banker who consulted for burning pains in his feet. Pains started approximately 6 months before referral, in both feet, slightly predominating in the right one. Pains were worse at night and increased on contact with the bed sheets. The patient could not sleep well and had to get up and walk around in the middle of the night. He measured 184cm and weighed 95kg. He had lost approximately 5kg voluntarily.

Upon examination muscle strength was normal. Temperature and pin-prick sensations were markedly decreased in the lower limbs, up to the mid-leg. Light touch was decreased over the feet. Position sense was normal. Vibratory sensation was abolished in the feet. The ankle reflexes were decreased. The upper limbs were normal as well as the rest of the neurological and general examination. His family history included type 2 diabetes in his father and elder brother.

EMG showed a marked decrease of sensory action potentials of sural nerves on both sides, with normal conduction velocity. Blood tests were normal with the exception of fasting blood sugar which was at 6.8mmol. Postprandial glucose was at 12mmol and glycosylated haemoglobin was 8.7%. The patient had blood tests done 2 years ago, which also had slightly abnormal sugar levels. The patient was treated with amitriptyline and was refered to a diabetologist.

In conclusion, this patient had type 2 diabetes of late onset, with an axonal polyneuropathy predominating on small fibres. Painful peripheral neuropathy is often the first and only clinical manifestation of type 2 diabetes.

Proximal diabetic neuropathy of the lower limbs

Louisa is a 55-year-old woman who had been treated for type 2 diabetes for 6 years. She was a little overweight, but in good general condition. Her diabetes was well controlled with a fasting glucose at 6.5mmol and glycosylated haemoglobin at 6.8%.

Two months before referral she started to complain of deep pain in the right thigh, which had gradually increased during the previous weeks. This became worse at night. The patient noticed spectacular wasting of the right thigh along with an increasing difficulty to climb stairs. Tight diabetic control with insulin did not help. She was treated with amitriptyline, and then with opiates. She had lost 6kg within 3 months. Neurological examination showed amyotrophy of the quadriceps muscle on the right side along with weakness of this muscle and of flexion of the hip. Distal strength was normal. She had sensory loss over the anterior aspect of the thigh and bilateral stocking hypoaesthesia. The patellar reflex was abolished on the right side. Magnetic resonance imaging (MRI) of the lumbar spine was normal. CSF examination showed 2.5g/L protein; there were no cells found.

In summary, this patient had a proximal neuropathy of the right lower limb in relation to type 2 diabetes.

After a few months the pain gradually disappeared and strength improved but she retained a marked amyotrophy of the right thigh.

Focal and multifocal neuropathy

Cranial nerve palsies improve spontaneously and do not require specific treatment. Proximal diabetic neuropathy is often very painful and should be treated with paracetamol and codeine, for example. Since some patients with disabling painful proximal neuropathy respond only to corticosteroids, this treatment should be considered in severe forms. This will require adjustment of diabetic control with insulin in most cases. Treatment of multifocal diabetic neuropathy is based on the use of corticosteroids for a few months. This requires adjustment of diabetic control.

Uraemic neuropathy

Introduction

Polyneuropathy is a potentially crippling disorder of patients on dialysis programmes, which can be prevented by early initiation of regular dialysis treatment and renal transplantation. In a few patients, however, it may still cause serious problems. The first report on uraemic neuropathy was made by Marin and Tyler in patients with hereditary interstitial nephritis with distal sensory motor polyneuropathy [27]. The term uraemic polyneuropathy was then used by Asbury *et al* [28].

Neuropathy generally only develops when glomerular filtration rates fall to 12ml/minute or below [29]. In most instances, both worsening and improvement evolve slowly over months, but on occasion neuropathy is fulminant in its course.

Symptoms and signs

Peripheral neuropathy is heralded by symptoms of dysfunction of lower motor neurons or of primary sensory neurons [30] (see case study on p124).

Muscle cramps and restless legs syndrome (RLS) have been considered to be symptoms of peripheral neuronal dysfunction in uraemic patients, but both symptoms actually lack specificity. Conversely, when patients complain of paraesthesias (tingling or prickling) in the toes, feet or fingers, clinical signs of uraemic neuropathy are usually present and may even be severe. Pain is absent in the early stages of neuropathy but may be prominent in advanced and severe neuropathy. Depressed or abolished ankle reflexes and an impaired vibration perception of the toes are early and initially the only clinical signs of peripheral neuropathy. Perception of light touch over distal lower limbs is affected first. In a minority of patients, neuropathy progresses further. Atrophy and weakness of distal leg muscles may develop as well as disturbance of all sensory modalities in a stocking-like distribution. Clinical signs of neuropathy in the upper limbs occur only in severe cases, even though alterations of

Uraemic neuropathy

Alice is a 63-year-old retired midday supervisor who had suffered with hypertension for 20 years and mature-onset diabetes mellitus for 9 years. She had had gradually failing renal function. Her glomerular filtration rate (eGFR) had been approximately 30ml/minute for the last couple of years, but she had failed to attend for her usual reviews for about 6 months. She presented with painful cold feet with a dysaesthetic component. Examination revealed a loss of light touch, vibration and pain perception in her toes, and her ankle reflexes were absent. Her peripheral neuropathy was initially attributed to her diabetes, which had been poorly controlled. Her eGFT came back at 10ml/minute, however. She was referred to the renal service and started on thrice-weekly haemodialysis. Within 3 months of starting dialysis her abnormal sensations in the feet had resolved; however, her loss of vibration perception and her ankle jerks did not return.

conduction velocity are present in all four limbs. Manifestations of autonomic neuropathy including postural hypotension, impaired sweating, diarrhoea, constipation, or impotence are usually not clinically manifest.

Nerve conduction slowing occurs to almost the same degree in motor and sensory nerve fibres, in nerves of upper and lower limbs and in proximal and distal parts of limb nerves. In the most severe cases conduction may fall to 60 or 50% of the normal values. Electrophysiological studies should be limited to patients who manifest symptoms of neuropathy. A significant decrease of the sensory action potential means that the patient has lost a significant proportion of large myelinated fibres in the nerve studied. The positive neuropathic symptoms correlate with quantitative vibratory detection thresholds and sensory nerve conduction studies, especially the amplitude of the sensory nerve action potential in the sural nerve [31].

Carpal tunnel syndrome (CTS) is a frequent complication of long-term haemodialysis. Twenty to 50% of patients dialysed for 10 years or longer are reported to have CTS. In most cases, the median nerve will be compressed by amyloid deposition or by the same factors that occur in non-uraemic individuals. In this situation, which is by far the most common, the preferred management is with surgical carpal tunnel release. Care must be taken to obtain a biopsy specimen of the flexor retinaculum to determine the presence of amyloid. Occasionally, the CTS may be related to the presence of an arteriovenous fistula in the forearm and can be managed by closure of the fistula.

Neuropathy and the degree of renal insufficiency

In patients regularly controlled in outpatient departments, signs of neuropathy are generally lacking as long as the creatinine clearance exceeds 60ml/minute. Successful kidney transplantation is followed by a two-phase course of recovery of neuropathy. The first phase is brief and begins within a few days after transplantation. Nerve conduction velocity increases and clinical signs rapidly improve. The second phase occurs slowly and lasts many months and results from axonal regeneration. Full clinical recovery occurs in most patients and nerve conduction may attain normal levels, although persistence of some delay of conduction, particularly in lower limb nerves, is not unusual.

Uraemic neuropathy in diabetic patients

In diabetic patients with renal insufficiency under dialysis treatment, the occurrence of severe axonal, length-dependent, sensory and motor polyneuropathy is common. In such patients it is virtually impossible to ascribe with certainty specific signs or symptoms to one or to the other metabolic disturbance. However, severe symptomatic autonomic disturbances, pain, and a length-dependent pattern of a loss of temperature and pain sensation, point to the predominant involvement of small myelinated and unmyelinated fibres, and are more characteristic of diabetic neuropathy [32]. Conversely, a prominent motor deficit is indicative of a predominant role for uraemia. After renal transplantation, the peripheral deficit which is related to uraemia would be anticipated to improve.

In conclusion, uraemic neuropathy can now be prevented by early and improved periodic haemodialysis and renal transplantation.

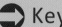 **Key points**

- Diabetic neuropathy is the most common neuropathy in the world.

- Distal symmetrical sensory polyneuropathy of insidious onset is the most common pattern of diabetic neuropathy. It often reveals type 2 diabetes of mature onset.

- Pain and trophic lesions in the foot (arthropathy and plantar ulcers) due to sensory denervation are common.

- Autonomic neuropathy can induce impotence, postural hypotension and diarrhoea.

- Diabetic oculomotor nerve palsies are spontaneously and completely reversible.

- Proximal neuropathy of the lower limbs is usually painful and disabling, with a self-limiting course.

- Uraemic neuropathy must be prevented by early periodic haemodialysis and renal transplantation.

References

1. International Diabetes Federation. IDF Diabetes Atlas, 6th edn. Brussels, Belgium: International Diabetes Federation, 2013. http://www.idf.org/diabetesatlas.

2. Pirart J. Diabetes mellitus and its degenerative complications: a prospective study of 4400 patients observed between 1947 and 1973. *Diabetes Care* 1978; 1: 168-88, 253-63.

3. Harris M, Eastman R, Cowie C. Symptoms of sensory neuropathy in adults with NIDDM in the U.S. population. *Diabetes Care* 1993; 16: 1446-52.

4. Young RJ, Zhou YQ, Rodriguez E, *et al*. Variable relationship between peripheral somatic and autonomic neuropathy in patients with different syndromes of diabetic polyneuropathy. *Diabetes* 1986; 35: 192-7.

5. Vergely P. Des troubles de la sensibilité aux membres inférieurs chez les diabétiques. De la dissociation syringomyélique de la sensibilité chez les diabétiques. *Gazette Hebdomadaire de Médecine et de Chirurgie* 1893; 32: 376-81.

6. Said G, Slama G, Selva J. Progressive centripetal degeneration of axons in small fibre type diabetic polyneuropathy. A clinical and pathological study. *Brain* 1983; 106: 791-807.

7. Charcot JM. Sur un cas de paraplégie diabétique. *Arch Neurol (Paris)* 1890; 19: 305-30.

8. Ellenberg M. Diabetic neuropathic cachexia. *Diabetes* 1974; 23: 418.

9. Archer AG, Watkins PJ, Thomas PK, *et al*. The natural history of acute painful neuropathy in diabetes mellitus. *J Neurol Neurosurg Psychiatry* 1983; 46: 491-9.

10. Llewelyn JG, Thomas PK, Fonseca V, *et al*. Acute painful diabetic neuropathy precipitated by strict glycaemic control. *Acta Neuropathol* 1986; 72: 157-63.

11. Lavery L, Armstrong D, Wunderlich R, *et al*. Diabetic foot syndrome: evaluating the prevalence and incidence of foot pathology in Mexican Americans and non-Hispanic whites from a diabetes disease management cohort. *Diabetes Care* 2003; 26: 1435.

12. Rundles RW. Diabetic neuropathy: general review with report of 125 cases. *Medicine (Baltimore)* 1945; 24: 111-60.

13. Bruns L. Ueber neuritische Lähmungen beim diabetes mellitus. *Berl Klin Wochenscher* 1890; 27: 509-15.

14. Asbury AK. Proximal diabetic neuropathy. *Ann Neurol* 1977; 2: 179.

15. Raff MC, Sangalang V, Asbury AK. Ischemic mononeuropathy and mononeuropathy multiplex in diabetes mellitus. *Arch Neurol* 1968; 18: 487-99.

16. Garland HT. Diabetic amyotrophy. *Br Med J* 1955; 2: 1287-90.

17. Coppack SW, Watkins PJ. The natural history of diabetic femoral neuropathy. *Q J Med* 1991; 79: 307-13.

18. Said G, Goulon-Goeau C, Lacroix C, *et al*. Nerve biopsy findings in different patterns of proximal diabetic neuropathy. *Ann Neurol* 1994; 35: 559-69.

19. Gavric M, Drulovic J, Stoisavlievic N, *et al*. Treatment with diabetic amotrophy with steroids. *Srp Arh Celok Lek* 1997; 125: 51-3.

20. Said G, Elgrably F, Lacroix C, *et al*. Painful proximal diabetic neuropathy: inflammatory nerve lesions and spontaneous favourable outcome. *Ann Neurol* 1997; 41: 762-70.

21. Ellenberg M. Diabetic truncal mononeuropathy: a new clinical syndrome. *Diabetes Care* 1978; 1: 10-3.

22. Said G, Lacroix C, Lozeron P, *et al*. Inflammatory vasculopathy in multifocal diabetic neuropathy. *Brain* 2003; 126: 376-85.

23. Cornblath D, Drachman DB, Griffin JW. Demyelinating motor neuropathy in patients with diabetic polyneuropathy. *Ann Neurol* 1987; 22: 126-32.

24. Stewart JD, McKelvey R, Durcan L, *et al*. Chronic inflammatory demyelinating polyneuropathy (CIDP) in diabetics. *J Neurol Sci* 1996; 142: 59-64.

25. Said G. Diabetic neuropathy. *Handb Clin Neurol* 2013; 115: 579-89.

26. Vincent AM, Calabek B, Roberts L, *et al.* Biology of diabetic neuropathy. *Handb Clin Neurol* 2013; 115: 591-606.

27. Marin OSM, Tyler HR. Hereditary interstitial nephritis associated with polyneuropathy. *Neurology (Minneap)* 1961; 11: 999-1005.

28. Asbury AK, Victor M, Adams RD. Uraemic polyneuropathy. *Arch Neurol* 1963; 8: 413-28.

29. Brouns R, De Deyn PP. Neurological complications in renal failure: a review. *Clin Neurol Neurosurg* 2004; 107: 1-16.

30. Bolton CF. Peripheral neuropathies associated with chronic renal failure. *Can J Neurol Sci* 1980; 7: 89-96.

31. Laaksonen S, Metsärinne K, Voipio-Pulkki LM, Falck B. Neurophysiologic parameters and symptoms in chronic renal failure. *Muscle Nerve* 2002; 25: 884-90.

32. Said G, Goulon-Goeau C, Slama G, *et al.* Severe early-onset polyneuropathy in insulin-dependent diabetes mellitus - a clinical and pathological study. *N Engl J Med* 1992; 326: 1257-63.

Chapter 9

Neuropathies in patients with monoclonal gammopathy and malignancy

Overview

In developed countries just under half of us will develop cancer at some stage in our lives and half the people who get cancer will live with the disease for more than 10 years. A number of cancers are associated with peripheral neuropathy. In addition, the treatment of cancer can be associated with the development of neuropathy. This chapter discusses the manifestations of neuropathy associated with cancer and related conditions.

Introduction

Monoclonal gammopathy is a condition whereby abnormal proteins are found in the blood. These proteins develop from a small number of plasma cells in the bone marrow. The most common condition linked with these abnormal proteins is monoclonal gammopathy of undetermined significance (MGUS). MGUS is not cancer, but rather a premalignant plasma cell disorder which is present in more than 3% of the general population aged over 50 years [1, 2]. People with MGUS have an increased risk of developing serious diseases of the bone marrow and blood.

Monoclonal gammopathy is often associated with polyneuropathy. As monoclonal gammopathy can be benign or associated with a malignant process, we have included both conditions in this chapter.

Malignant conditions may have a direct effect upon peripheral nerves by invasion of roots or nerve trunks by malignant cells, or a remote effect through paraneoplastic manifestations. Also, treatment of cancer by chemotherapy or by irradiation may have a deleterious effect on the peripheral nervous system (PNS).

Neuropathy and monoclonal gammopathy

Benign monoclonal gammopathy

Benign monoclonal gammopathy can be associated with chronic inflammatory demyelinating polyneuropathy (CIDP). This is often the case for the immunoglobulin M (IgM) kappa monoclonal gammopathy. Antibodies directed against the myelin-associated glycoprotein (MAG) are often associated with IgM monoclonal gammopathy and polyneuropathy. The picture and course of the neuropathy is very similar to that of CIDP, but yearly review of the gammopathy is necessary due to the possible malignant transformation occurring in this setting.

Monoclonal gammopathy and light chain amyloidosis

Monoclonal gammopathy (mostly IgG) can also be associated with light chain amyloidosis. This disorder is suspected in patients who develop a subacute progressive length-dependent sensory and motor polyneuropathy associated with serious autonomic manifestations and carpal tunnel syndrome. Cardiac manifestations, including an intracardiac conduction defect and cardiac failure, are common manifestations in this condition. The diagnosis rests on demonstration of amyloid deposits in tissue biopsy and exclusion of a hereditary form of amyloidosis (Figure 1).

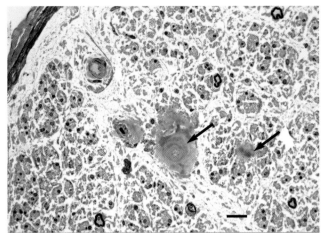

Figure 1. Nerve biopsy from a patient with monoclonal gammopathy and a severe sensory-motor polyneuropathy due to light chain amyloidosis. Endoneurial amyloid deposits are illustrated by arrows. Note the nearly complete disappearance of nerve fibres, in keeping with this severe neuropathy. (Bar 10µm.)

The POEMS syndrome (polyneuropathy, organomegaly, endocrinopathy, monoclonal gammopathy, skin changes)

POEMS syndrome is a rare multisystem disease associated with plasma cell dyscrasia [3]. POEMS is defined by the association of peripheral neuropathy and a monoclonal plasma cell disorder with other systemic features including organomegaly (splenomegaly, hepatomegaly, or lymphadenopathy), endocrinopathy (adrenal, thyroid, pituitary, severe diabetes, gonadal, and others), and skin changes (particularly hyperpigmentation, acrocyanosis, white nails, hypertrichosis, and haemangiomata). Peripheral oedema, pleural effusions or ascites, pulmonary hypertension, renal involvement (mesangiocapillary-like glomerulonephritis), papilloedema, thrombocytosis, and polycythemia also occur in this syndrome. Virtually all patients have either at least one sclerotic bone lesion (rarely lytic lesions) or coexistent Castleman disease (Figure 2). Monoclonal proteins are usually IgG or IgA and almost invariably bear the lambda light chain. Their level is often quite low. The

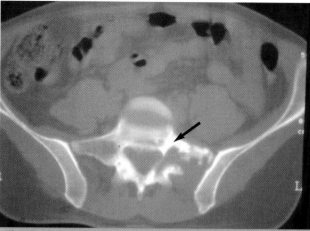

Figure 2. CT scan of the sacrum showing a sclerotic bone lesion (arrow) in a patient with POEMS syndrome.

neuropathy in POEMS is quite severe and often presents subacutely and is often rapidly disabling. It is predominantly a motor neuropathy, frequently starting with sensory symptoms. Often, patients are initially diagnosed with CIDP due to the subacute progression in terms of months and the prominent demyelinating features on nerve conduction studies (Figure 3). Plasma and serum levels of vascular endothelial growth factor (VEGF) are markedly elevated in patients with POEMS and correlate with the activity of the disease and response to therapy. Irradiation or surgical excision remain the therapy of choice for patients with dominant sclerotic plasmacytoma [3], while patients with diffuse lesions or disseminated bone marrow involvement should undergo systemic chemotherapy.

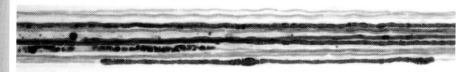

Figure 3. Teased fibre preparation from a nerve biopsy of a patient with POEMS syndrome, showing demyelination of nerve fibres.

Malignant cell infiltration of the PNS

Infiltration of the PNS by malignant cells is relatively rare, compared to neuropathies related to toxicity of medications used to treat malignant disorders, or to radiation-induced nerve lesions. Malignant cell infiltration more commonly affects spinal roots than peripheral nerves. Infiltration of the PNS within the subarachnoid space occurs in leukaemia and in different types of carcinoma (Figure 4). A multifocal sensory-motor deficit, affecting several root territories, may be the initial and only symptomatic manifestation of cancer. Magnetic resonance imaging (MRI) of spinal roots may show multiple small tumours, and cerebrospinal fluid (CSF) examination reveals a high protein content with low glucose and the presence of malignant cells. Subarachnoid chemotherapy often gives good results [4].

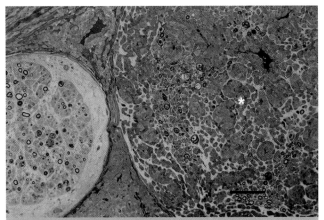

Figure 4. Nerve biopsy findings in a patient with plasma cell leukaemia and relapsing multifocal neuropathy. Note the massive infiltration of malignant plasma cells in the nerve fascicle (asterisk). (Bar 50µm.)

Invasion of the brachial plexus occurs in patients with carcinoma of the lung, sometimes on both sides (Pancoast tumour). This invasion of the PNS also may occur in association with lymphomas (➲ see case study overleaf) and sometimes is the initial manifestation of lymphoma as

Demyelinating polyneuropathy

Mohammed is a 31-year-old security guard who developed a swelling in the left side of his neck. He was investigated and found to have widespread lymphadenopathy. A biopsy was undertaken and misinterpreted as showing changes consistent with a diagnosis of tuberculosis (TB). He was started on quadruple therapy of isoniazid, rifampicin, pyrazinamide and ethambutol with pyridoxine 10mg a day. He developed painful feet and by the time he was admitted to hospital he could not walk. Initially, consideration was given to a drug-induced neuropathy. The diagnosis was reviewed and a further biopsy demonstrated lymphoma. Peripheral neurophysiology showed changes consistent with a demyelinating polyneuropathy. Within a month of commencing his chemotherapy for his lymphoma his neuropathy had started to improve. By 6 months after the initiation of chemotherapy he was able to walk, albeit unsteadily. After 3 years, he remains free of lymphoma, but he has a loss of pain perception in his feet as well as a loss of vibration sense and proprioception. There is wasting and weakness of the muscles in his lower legs. He has significant persistent neuropathic pain. He remains unemployed.

in neurolymphomatosis, which is associated with monoclonal gammopathy.

Paraneoplastic neuropathies

Paraneoplastic syndromes affect the PNS in up to one third of patients with solid tumours. The classic syndrome consists of a subacute sensory neuronopathy. However, other variations in the rate of progression of neuropathy, pattern of neuropathy, degree of sensory, motor, and autonomic involvement, and the presence or absence of specific onconeural antibodies can occur [5].

The term 'onconeural antibodies' (paraneoplastic antibodies) applies to antibodies that target antigens present in nervous tissue and tumours, thus paraneoplastic neurological syndromes could be the result of an immunological response triggered against tumoural antigens and misdirected to similar antigens expressed in the nervous system. Small-cell lung cancer is the common cause of paraneoplastic peripheral neuropathy, but it is also seen in lymphoma, breast, and gynaecological cancers, and thymoma.

Subacute sensory neuronopathy is caused by damage to sensory neurons in the dorsal root ganglia (ganglionopathy). Symptoms evolve in days to a few weeks. The predominant complaints at the onset are pain and paraesthesias, with an asymmetrical distribution that involves the arms rather than the legs. Numbness, limb ataxia, and pseudoathetotic movements of the hands are often observed. The tendon reflexes are lost and all modalities of sensation are involved but with a clear predominance of joint position and vibratory sense. The face can be affected due to trigeminal ganglia damage. Sensorineural deafness and sensory deficits in the trunk are unusual. The typical sensory neuronopathy has a subacute evolution which subsequently stabilizes. By the time it does so, however, the patient is usually confined to a bed or chair due to ataxia [6]. In 10% of patients, the neuropathy runs a mild and very slow clinical evolution. These patients may remain ambulatory and independent for years. The specificity and sensitivity of anti-Hu antibodies is high. Only 18% of patients with a paraneoplastic sensory neuronopathy were Hu-Ab negative. Small-cell lung cancer was the leading neoplasm in the Hu-positive (79%) and Hu-negative (44%) groups [7]. Patients without anti-Hu antibodies may harbour CV2 or amphiphysin antibodies. Other paraneoplastic neuropathies include less common manifestations such as sensory-motor neuropathy, autonomic neuropathy and chronic intestinal pseudo-obstruction.

Neuropathy in patients treated for malignant disorders

In addition to lesions of the PNS due to invasion by malignant cells or to paraneoplastic syndromes, patients with cancer are exposed to complications linked to chemotherapy or to radiation.

Post-radiation neuropathies

Peripheral neuropathies are rare, late complications of radiation therapy. The most frequent form and the best understood peripheral nerve damage due to radiation is brachial plexopathy, which complicates irradiation for breast cancer. The time to onset ranges from several months to decades with a mean incidence of 1.8-2.9% per year. The incidence of radiation-induced brachial plexopathy today is under 1-2% in patients receiving usual plexus total doses of less than 55Gy in 2Gy daily fractions. Radiation-induced brachial plexopathy (RIBP) varies greatly in intensity, but gradual worsening over several years may result in paralysis of the upper limb with a mean time of 1.2 years (range 0.2-5) from the first symptoms to hand paralysis. Skin changes, especially poikilodermia, are associated with induration of the axillary-subclavicular area with subcutaneous fibrosis, advanced osteoporosis, and even sternoclavicular osteonecrosis with, in older female patients, subcutaneous calcification. Lymphoedema occurs in approximately 20% of cases in some series. Electromyography (EMG) is useful in this setting. Also, MRI of the brachial plexus is needed to exclude invasion of the brachial plexus by the cancer itself.

Lumbosacral radiculoplexopathy is less common than brachial plexopathy. The interval between irradiation and symptom onset ranges between 1 and 30 years after irradiation for testicular cancer or lymphomas. Motor deficit predominates. Damage of the surrounding tissues is frequently associated with radiculoplexus damage. Only symptomatic treatment is available for post-radiation nerve lesions.

Post-chemotherapy peripheral neuropathy

Drugs used to treat malignant disorders are among the most frequent causes of toxic neuropathy [8]. In addition, most of these neuropathies are preventable by appropriate monitoring.

Chemotherapy-induced peripheral neuropathy (CIPN) is a major dose-limiting side effect of many of the commonly used agents, including platinum compounds (cisplatin and carboplatin), taxanes (paclitaxel), and vinca alkaloids (vincristine). Newer agents such as bortezomib, lenalidomide, ixabepilone, and the newest platinum compound, oxaliplatin, also have significant neuropathic side effects.

Vinca alkaloids

Vincristine sulfate and vincaleucoblastine are commonly used in the treatment of haematological and lymphatic malignancies, as well as in the treatment of some solid tumours of the breast and lung. Commonly used combination regimens include CHOP (cyclophosphamide, hydroxydaunorubicin, Oncovin® [vincristine], and prednisolone) and MOPP (mechlorethamine, Oncovin®, procarbazine, and prednisolone). Reduced or absent ankle reflexes occur in most patients treated with vincristine. Muscle weakness, which may develop rapidly over about 10 days, involves the toe and ankle dorsiflexors as well as plantarflexors, and in severe cases the finger and wrist extensors. Autonomic dysfunction with abdominal pain, constipation, paralytic ileus and bladder atony can occur. Recovery is usually over the course of a few weeks.

Platinum compounds

These include cisplatin, oxaliplatin and carboplatin. Cisplatin is a first-line treatment for testicular cancer — the most common form of cancer in men between the ages of 15 and 35 years. It has resulted in a cure rate of more than 80%. In addition, it is also used as adjunctive therapy in cancers of the lung, bladder, oesophagus, head and neck, and cervix. It is the most commonly used chemotherapeutic agent in the USA. A severe oxaliplatin neuropathy occurs in 10-20% of patients at a cumulative dose of 750mg/m² and in 50% at higher doses.

Carboplatin is now the first-line drug for ovarian cancer but it is also used in breast cancer, often in combination with paclitaxel, and in metastatic lung cancer. It seems less neurotoxic than cisplatin but will cause a similar neuropathy at higher doses. Oxaliplatin, a third-generation organoplatin compound, is used in advanced or metastatic colorectal cancer. All platinum compounds can induce a sensory neuropathy mainly affecting large fibres, with sensory ataxia often with Lhermitte's phenomenon (suggestive of posterior column involvement). Oxaliplatin causes, in 95% of patients, an acute syndrome of severe cold hypersensitivity, jaw tightness, cramps, and perioral, pharyngeal and limb paraesthesias soon after infusion which resolves within hours or days.

Taxanes

Paclitaxel is used alone or in combination for the treatment of ovarian cancer, metastatic breast cancer, and non-small-cell lung cancer. The neuropathy induced is similar but milder than the vinca alkaloid neuropathy, but it can be dose-limiting.

Thalidomide

In recent years, thalidomide has become incorporated into treatment regimens either in combination with high-dose dexamethasone, in preparation for autologous transplantation, or with low-dose melphalan and prednisolone in elderly or frail patients. Thalidomide induces a large fibre length-dependent toxic polyneuropathy if not stopped at the first manifestation of toxicity. Therefore, close monitoring of these patients is mandatory. The administration of thalidomide must be interrupted if perception of light touch (cotton) is decreased in the feet, or if there is a significant decrease in sural nerve sensory action potentials.

Bortezomid

The neuropathy caused by bortezomid (a proteasome inhibitor) is a length-dependent sensory neuropathy affecting small fibres, often causing significant neuropathic pain. In up to 30%, dose modification or cessation of treatment may be necessary.

Drug-induced polyneuropathy is a real burden in patients with cancer and a major limiting factor for chemotherapy. In some patients cured from cancer, sequelae of toxic polyneuropathy remain a major complaint and factor of disability.

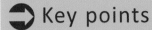 **Key points**

- Benign IgM monoclonal gammopathy is often associated with a demyelinating polyneuropathy.
- POEMS syndrome (polyneuropathy, organomegaly, endocrinopathy, monoclonal gammopathy, and skin changes) with increased levels of VEGF, responds well to treatment of the plasma cell proliferation.
- Malignant infiltration of the PNS is usually restricted to spinal roots.
- Small-cell lung cancer is the most common cause of subacute sensory paraneoplastic neuronopathy and is usually associated with anti-Hu antibodies.
- Radiotherapy and chemotherapy for cancer can both induce peripheral nerve damage, which should be prevented by appropriate monitoring.

References

1. Kyle RA, Therneau TM, Rajkumar SV, *et al*. Prevalence of monoclonal gammopathy of undetermined significance. *N Engl J Med* 2006; 354(13): 1362-9.
2. Kyle RA, Durie BGM, Rajkumar SV, *et al*. Monoclonal gammopathy of undetermined significance (MGUS) and smoldering (asymptomatic) multiple myeloma: IMWG consensus perspectives risk factors for progression and guidelines for monitoring and management. *Leukemia* 2010; 24(6): 1121-7.
3. Dispenzieri A. POEMS syndrome: 2011 update on diagnosis, risk-stratification, and management. *Am J Hematol* 2011; 86: 592-601.
4. Grisold W, Briani C, Vass A. Malignant cell infiltration in the peripheral nervous system. *Handb Clin Neurol* 2013; 115: 685-712.
5. Giometto B, Grisold W, Vitaliani R, *et al*. Paraneoplastic neurological syndrome in the PNS Euronetwork database: a European study from 20 centres. *Arch Neurol* 2010; 67: 330-5.
6. Graus F, Keime-Guibert F, Rene R, *et al*. Anti-Hu associated paraneoplastic encephalomyelitis: analysis of 200 patients. *Brain* 2001; 124: 1138-48.

7. Molinuevo JL, Graus F, Serrano C, *et al.* Utility of anti-Hu antibodies in the diagnosis of paraneoplastic sensory neuropathy. *Ann Neurol* 1998; 44: 976-80.

8. Manji H. Drug-induced neuropathies. *Handb Clin Neurol* 2013; 115: 729-42.

Chapter 10

Hereditary neuropathies

Overview

This chapter deals with neuropathies that are genetically transmitted. Predominantly motor hereditary neuropathy with the classic Charcot-Marie-Tooth disease, now encompasses several distinct phenotypes and genotypes, axonal or demyelinating, with a dominant or recessive transmission. Predominantly sensory and autonomic neuropathies include several clinical and pathological patterns which can be restricted to the peripheral nervous system, or associated with life-threatening polysystemic manifestations as in amyloid polyneuropathies and Fabry's disease. Treatment of these conditions is outlined. Genetic counselling is mandatory in these life-threatening hereditary disorders.

Introduction

For almost a century after the description of the dominantly transmitted motor and sensory neuropathies described by Charcot, Marie, and Tooth, subsequently known as Charcot-Marie-Tooth disease (CMT), and the recessive, early-onset neuropathy described by Dejerine and Sottas, the field remained virtually unchanged until the classification of CMT disease following nerve conduction studies. More recently, progress in molecular genetics has led to the discovery of a variety of different hereditary neuropathies. Besides the classical CMT disease, which now encompasses several distinct phenotypes and genotypes, hereditary neuropathies include a variety of sensory and autonomic neuropathies.

Another group of hereditary neuropathies are associated with life-threatening polysystemic manifestations as in amyloid polyneuropathies, Fabry's disease, neuropathies associated with mitochondriopathies, to name but a few. Each of these diseases can be related to several DNA mutations. Thus, DNA testing is now a major step in the diagnosis and management of hereditary neuropathies, but in all instances DNA testing must be oriented by the clinical pattern and family history. The complexity of familial polyneuropathy makes it advisable to refer patients with suspected or confirmed familial neuropathy to expert centres where they can get the best advice. First we will consider the Charcot-Marie-Tooth group, which is historically the first described, predominantly motor and typically carrying an autosomal dominant transmission. Where we once thought of CMT disease as a homogeneous entity, there are now something like 50 different mutations which can induce the same phenotype, with some variants.

Hereditary neuropathies without polysystemic manifestations

Predominantly motor hereditary polyneuropathies

Two main patterns have been originally identified: the CMT pattern, which is the most common, is benign and dominantly transmitted. The other one is an early-onset, recessively transmitted phenotype, which corresponds to Dejerine-Sottas disease.

Late onset and dominant transmission

The Charcot-Marie-Tooth neuropathies [1]

The typical CMT phenotype is characterised by onset in the first decades of life, of slowly progressive bilateral muscle wasting and weakness starting with the feet and legs and then gradually ascending to the distal third of the thigh and hands. Sensory loss is less prominent, and pains are usually mild or absent. Sensory changes follow the same distribution as motor changes. Skeletal foot deformities are very common: pes cavus with high arches and hammer toes is found in the majority of affected subjects since childhood (Figure 1). Scoliosis is present in one third of patients. Upon examination, motor deficit, which starts and predominates in the distal foot, is mild and progresses very slowly, over decades. Most patients remain able to walk, although with increasing difficulty and they often need special shoes. Deep tendon reflexes are absent from the onset. CMT disease, however, is characterised by a high variability of disease severity including within the same family. In some members the expression of the disease is limited to pes cavus, while in others foot deformity is associated with foot drop after a few decades. Some affected patients may be confined to a wheelchair, with severe loss of hand movements.

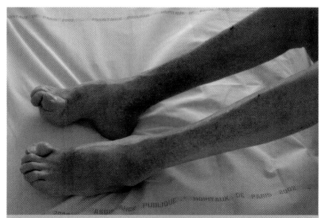

Figure 1. Pes cavus and leg amyotrophy in a patient with a Charcot-Marie-Tooth hereditary neuropathy and PMP22 duplication.

The subdivision into two main types according to nerve conduction studies, was a cornerstone in the CMT nosography and is still valid in the majority of cases. CMT1 designates the demyelinating variety and is characterised by diffuse slowing of nerve conduction velocities (NCV), with values by convention below the limit of 38m/second for motor nerves in the upper limbs. CMT2 is the axonal type, in which NCVs are preserved, or only mildly slowed, by definition above the value of 38m/second in upper limb motor nerves.

Within the CMT phenotype, DNA testing has identified some subclasses as outlined below.

CMT1

CMT1A is related to duplication of the 17p peripheral myelin protein 22 (*PMP22*), or less often to *PMP22* point mutation. CMT1A accounts for 60-90% of CMT1 patients (◐ see case study overleaf). In CMT1A patients, nerve biopsy shows extensive demyelination of nerve fibres associated

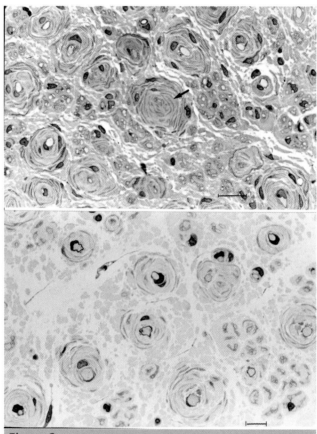

Figure 2. Cross-sections of a nerve biopsy specimen to show Schwann cell proliferation forming onion bulbs common in the hypertrophic type of demyelinating CMT disease. (Bar 10μm.)

with spectacular proliferation of Schwann cells which may induce palpable nerve hypertrophy (Figure 2).

Charcot-Marie-Tooth disease type 1

Charles is a 53-year-old physiotherapist who consulted because of walking difficulty. The patient was in good general condition and worked in a rehabilitation centre in a university hospital. He first noticed some difficulty in walking 2 to 3 years previously, in that he would become fatigued after walking for an hour or two. This fatigue gradually increased over the subsequent years to the point where he had to rest after walking for half an hour. Upon examination he had bilateral pes cavus and hammer toes, and said that he always had problems to find convenient shoes. His legs were slightly atrophic distally. He had no pain. He could not stand on the heels on either side. The strength of foot dorsiflexion was decreased to 4/5 and plantar flexion was normal. Muscle strength was normal in other territories. Perception of light touch was abolished up to the mid-leg, but pinprick and temperature sensations were preserved. Position sense of the great toe was decreased on both sides. Ankle and patellar reflexes were abolished.

With regard to family history, the patient had a 48-year-old sister who had no walking difficulties. The patient's mother, who was 82 years old, had marked walking difficulty which had necessitated the use of a walking cane since the age of 75. Her younger sister who was 67 years old had bilateral pes cavus but no walking difficulty. An electromyography (EMG) showed a reduced nerve conduction velocity in the upper and lower limbs. Peroneal nerve conduction was reduced to 24m/s on the right side; 22m/s on the left side with an important decrease of the compound muscle action potentials. In the upper limbs, the median nerve conduction velocity was 28m/s on both sides. DNA testing for dominant demyelinating Charcot-Marie-Tooth disease confirmed that the patient had duplication of the 17p peripheral myelin protein 22 gene.

This patient had a relatively mild expression of the disease. This mutation had a variable expression amongst his relatives. The patient's aunt only had pes cavus and the patient's mother was still able to walk.

CMT1B is related to mutation of the myelin P zero protein (*MPZ*) gene. CMT1B accounts for approximately 10% of CMT1. The phenotype of patients with *MPZ* mutations is usually one of two types, an early-onset neuropathy with slow motor NCV, which can be severe — as in the Dejerine-Sottas syndrome — or an adult-onset, milder axonal or intermediate neuropathy. CMT1 C, D, E and F are rare demyelinating CMT types, accounting for less than 1% of CMT disease.

CMT2

CMT2 has the same clinical presentation and transmission as CMT1, but nerve conduction velocity is in the axonal pattern, in keeping with nerve pathology. The most common type is CMT2A related to mitofusin 2 mutation (*MFN2*)(*1p36.2 MFN2*). It accounts for up to 20% of the

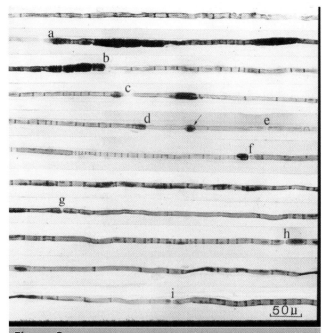

Figure 3. Consecutive segments of an isolated nerve fibre from a patient with an hereditary liability to pressure palsy, showing the thickness variation of the myelin sheath with a 'sausage' formation.

CMT2 group, which may be either severe with an early onset or mild to moderate with a later onset. There are frequent *de novo* mutations. The CMT2B to P types are much rarer and related to a variety of mutations.

CMTX1

The X-linked dominant variety of CMT disease, CMTX1, is characterised by clinical and electrophysiological involvement more severe in males, who often have NCV in the intermediate range, than females, whose NCV are usually in the CMT2 range.

Hereditary neuropathy with a liability to pressure palsy (HNPP)

HNPP typically presents with recurrent transient focal motor and/or sensory deficits in the distribution of individual nerves or plexuses, usually precipitated by pressure. There is slowing at typical sites of compression. All patients with HNPP have widespread neurophysiological abnormalities even if their symptoms are confined to a single nerve [2]. HNPP is usually caused by deletion of the same 1.4 Mb region of chromosome 17 that is duplicated in CMT1A. Nerve biopsy shows characteristic swelling of the myelin sheath called tomacula (Figure 3).

Recessive transmission of early-onset CMT neuropathies and the Dejerine-Sottas phenotype

Autosomal recessive cases are rare in Europe, accounting for less than 10% of CMT patients. Conversely, this inheritance pattern is frequent in populations with a high rate of consanguineous marriages as in North Africa and Turkey [3]. Dejerine-Sottas syndrome splits into the autosomal recessive CMT4 phenotypes. The recessively transmitted CMT syndromes have in common an early onset, within the first years of life, delayed developmental milestones and a severe outcome.

Recessive demyelinating neuropathy — CMT4A

CMT4A onset is in the first decade of life and the progression is rapid and severe. Classical features of CMT disease, like distal weakness and wasting, reduced or abolished reflexes, and pes cavus are often accompanied by proximal involvement and very early paralysis of the hands. Patients are usually wheelchair-bound late in the disease progression, yet the severity of the disease may vary among affected individuals in the same family with the same mutation. Special attention must be paid to these patients with investigation of respiratory function since it is life-threatening. CMT4A is associated with a variety of mutations in the *GDAP1* gene.

CMT4B1

The onset is usually before the age of 4 years. Weakness distribution is similar to the classical CMT phenotype; it starts distally in the lower limbs, then affects the upper limbs progressing to involve proximal muscles. Deep tendon reflexes are usually absent with distal sensory loss. A pes equinovarus deformity is reported in some patients. Patients are usually wheelchair-bound at an early age. Cranial nerve involvement is reported. Causative mutation occurs in the myotubularin-related protein 2 gene (*MTMR2*). The CMT4C to CMT4J types are rare, with an early or very early onset, or at birth. These are demyelinating polyneuropathies with a recessive transmission, related to a variety of rare mutations, sometimes affecting a single family.

To summarise the genetic findings in patients with CMT disease, it is of interest to quote the findings of an important study of 425 patients. The study consisted of 240 patients with CMT1 (56%), 115 with CMT2 (27%) and 62 with CMT disease associated with intermediately slowed nerve conduction (ICMT). Ninety-two percent of those patients with CMT disease and a genetic diagnosis had either a duplication of *PMP22* (CMT1A) or mutations in three other genes; *MPZ* (CMT1B), gap junction beta-1 (*GJB1* — CMT1X) or *MFN2* (CMT2A). If no mutation was detected with these four genes, there was less than a 3% chance of making a molecular diagnosis. This was true of course only for patients with autosomal dominant or X-linked CMT disease, although as the authors point out, many of these patients may present without a family history [4, 5].

Hereditary sensory and autonomic neuropathies

This group of hereditary neuropathies encompasses a variety of purely or predominantly sensory polyneuropathies that may or may not be associated with manifestations of dysautonomia. In this group too, some neuropathies are transmitted as an autosomal trait, often with a late onset, while at the other extremity of the spectrum, some neuropathies are symptomatic as early as during the first days of life.

Hereditary sensory and autonomic neuropathy type I

Hereditary sensory and autonomic neuropathy type I (HSN I/HSAN I) disease is an autosomal dominant genetic subtype. Its onset is usually between the second and fourth decade of life or even later when patients first notice marked distal sensory impairment in the lower but sometimes also the upper limbs. Variable distal motor and minimal autonomic involvement is frequently observed. The neurological phenotype is often complicated by painless injuries which lead to severe infection including deep foot ulceration, osteomyelitis and osteonecrosis, and acromutilations that may necessitate toe and limb amputation. Spontaneous lancinating pains are sometimes reported. So far, five genes (*SPTLC1*, *SPTLC2*, *RAB7A*, *ATL1*, and *DNMT1*) have been implicated in the pathogenesis of

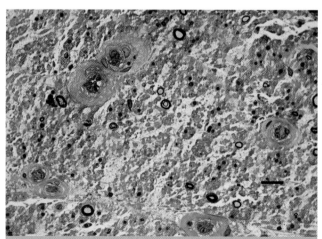

Figure 4. Cross-section of a nerve specimen from a patient with type 1 hereditary sensory and autonomic neuropathy. Light microscopy shows the nearly complete disappearance of myelinated fibres. (Bar 10µm.)

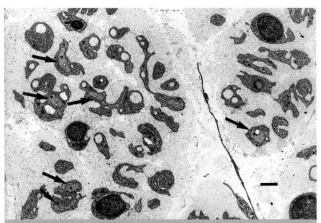

Figure 5. Electron micrograph of the same nerve specimen to show a spectacular reduction of the number of unmyelinated fibres. The surviving unmyelinated fibres are indicated by arrows. (Bar 1μm.)

HSN I. Electromyography (EMG) findings are characterised by decreased or absent sensory action potentials and relative preservation of nerve conduction velocity. From a pathological point of view this subtype is characterised by the gradual disappearance of myelinated and unmyelinated nerve fibres (Figures 4 and 5). The main complication of this subtype is the occurrence of distal trophic chances resulting from painless trauma. Phenotypic variability within a family varies widely and, also, subclinically affected mutation carriers have been described [6].

Hereditary sensory and autonomic neuropathy type II

Hereditary sensory and autonomic neuropathy type II (HSN II/HSAN II) is an autosomal recessively inherited form of HSN (see case study overleaf). At disease onset, patients usually show signs and symptoms consisting of distal numbness in the upper and lower limbs and a glove and stocking-like sensory loss in infancy or early childhood. Later on, patients develop impairment of pain, temperature and touch sensation,

Hereditary sensory neuropathy type II

Nelly is a 29-year-old woman who consulted for chronic sensory loss with recurrent corneal ulcers, multiple painless trauma, acral mutilation and painless burns during infancy and childhood. She was born to non-consanguineous parents. She had one older brother and one younger sister, none of whom were affected. She was married and a mother of a 3-year-old daughter who did not seem affected.

The patient was hypotrophic measuring 148cm and weighed 35kg. She had a scoliosis and delayed development milestones. She could not walk unaided until the age of 7 years. She had no symptoms of dysautonomia. She was an intelligent person. She had an ataxic gait, with normal motor strength. Sensory examination revealed a universal loss of pain and temperature sensation. She could not identify materials by palpation. Proprioception was abolished, including position sense, vibratory sensation and astereognosia. She had a sensory ataxia with Romberg's sign. All tendon reflexes were abolished. Electrophysiological testing showed normal motor action potentials and conduction velocity. The sensory action potentials were undetectable. A biopsy of the left sural nerve was performed which showed small nerve fascicles and nearly a complete absence of myelinated fibres. Conversely, the unmyelinated fibres were preserved (Figure 6).

This patient had a purely sensory polyneuropathy of early onset with dysmorphic changes, without autonomic dysfunction. This is a recessive autonomic hereditary sensory neuropathy type II associated with mutation in the *WNK1* gene, which was later confirmed by DNA testing. The patient was followed for several years without a significant change in her neurological condition.

involving the trunk in some patients as well. Autonomic dysfunction may be minimal and can include hyperhidrosis, tonic pupils, and urinary incontinence in cases with more advanced disease. At present, mutations in three genes (*HSN2/WNK1*, *FAM134B* and *KIF1A*) have been associated with HSN II phenotypes.

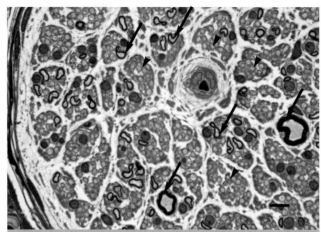

Figure 6. One-micron-thick cross-section of a plastic-embedded sural nerve biopsy specimen. Note the nearly complete absence of myelinated fibres (arrows) contrasting with the large number of unmyelinated axons (arrowheads). (Thionin blue staining. Bar: 5μm.)

Hereditary sensory and autonomic neuropathy type III — the Riley-Day syndrome

Hereditary sensory and autonomic neuropathy type III (HSN III/HSAN III) is an autosomal recessive developmental disorder affecting small myelinated and unmyelinated neurons resulting in sensory and autonomic dysfunction. Symptoms are present from birth with the earliest signs being poor suck and hypotonia. Clinical diagnostic criteria include absent lacrimation, absent deep tendon reflexes, and absent lingual fungiform papillae. Autonomic dysfunction results in absent emotional tears, oromotor incoordination, and cardiovascular lability with postural hypotension and episodic hypertension. Patients are also prone to periodic vomiting crises comprising nausea, hypersalivation, bronchorrhea, hypertension, tachycardia, and erythematous blotching of the skin. Familial dysautonomia is caused by mutations in the inhibitor of kappa light polypeptide gene enhancer in B-cells, kinase complex-associated protein (*IKBKAP*) gene which encodes a protein termed IKK complex-associated protein (IKAP); this gene is located in chromosome 9q31. A high frequency has been shown among Ashkenazi Jews [7].

Hereditary sensory and autonomic neuropathy type IV

Hereditary sensory and autonomic neuropathy type IV (HSN IV/HSAN IV) is also known as congenital insensitivity to pain and anhydrosis. Disease onset is at birth. HSAN IV is characterised by a congenital profound sensory loss affecting perception of pain and temperature, and an absence of sweating. Routine electrophysiological studies such as motor and sensory conduction velocities are usually normal. Histopathological findings consist of decreased numbers of unmyelinated and small myelinated fibres in sensory nerves (Figure 7).

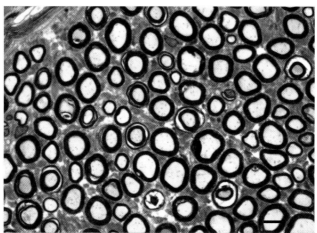

Figure 7. This nerve biopsy specimen from a patient with type IV hereditary sensory and autonomic neuropathy shows complete preservation of myelinated fibres. In this type of sensory neuropathy only the unmyelinated fibres are affected. (Bar: 10μm.)

Hereditary neuropathies with polysystemic manifestations

This is a group of life-threatening hereditary polyneuropathies due to severe polysystemic involvement including cardiac and renal manifestations. Enormous progress has been made in this field, not only on the genetic aspects but also on therapy, especially in familial amyloid polyneuropathy.

Familial amyloid polyneuropathies

Amyloidoses are a group of diseases characterised by tissue deposition of insoluble proteins and fibril aggregates oriented in a β-pleated sheet structure that form unbranched amyloid fibrils of 10-12nm diameter, which are deleterious to surrounding tissue. Amyloidosis can be acquired or hereditary. There are three main types of familial amyloid polyneuropathy (FAP), defined according to the precursor protein of amyloid: transthyretin (TTR) (➲ see case study overleaf), apolipoprotein A-1, and gelsolin [8-10]. The most common FAP is the one related to mutation of the transthyretin gene first reported in Portugal.

Mutated transthyretin-familial amyloid polyneuropathy (TTR-FAP)
FAP was first described by Andrade in 1952, in northern Portugal. The disease was also subsequently found to be endemic in Japan and Sweden. Eventually TTR-FAP was reported in a number of other countries.

Two main patterns of sensory-motor deficit occur in patients with TTR-FAP, both associated with variable autonomic disturbance and extra-neurological manifestations.

Length-dependent sensory-motor polyneuropathy
Typically the first symptoms of this type of polyneuropathy occur in adult patients in their mid-thirties in Portugal, and often after 50 years of age in Sweden, Japan and France. Symptoms start with discomfort over the feet, numbness and often pain. At this stage clinical examination can already detect an impaired thermal sensibility over the feet, with a decreased pin-prick sensation. Conversely, light touch and proprioception are preserved.

Late-onset transthyretin familial amyloid polyneuropathy

Susan, a 55-year-old female, had complained of hand numbness for the past 2 years, affecting first the right, then the left hand, with paraesthesias, loss of sensation of all fingers, and gradual wasting. She was in good general condition, with no significant family history for neurological disorders. Examination showed a loss of sensation of all fingers with muscle atrophy. Tendon reflexes were normal as was the rest of the neurological examination. Carpal tunnel syndrome was considered but all fingers were affected, which is uncommon in carpal tunnel syndrome as compression is normally restricted to the median nerve, with no overlap on the ulnar nerve territory.

Nerve conduction studies showed a loss of compound motor and sensory action potentials in both the median and ulnar nerve territories. There were normal findings in the lower limbs. The right sural nerve action potential was normal (11μV). Routine blood tests were normal. Carpal tunnel syndrome and ulnar compression were considered and surgery performed.

A year later the patient started to complain of burning pains in the feet associated with episodic diarrhoea and gradual weight loss. Neurological examination then showed a loss of pain and temperature sensation over the feet, up to the mid-leg. Light touch perception was decreased over the feet and proprioception was normal. There was a slight decrease of foot dorsiflexion. Ankle reflexes were abolished. In the upper limbs, temperature sensation was impaired up to the mid-forearm.

Nerve conduction studies showed a marked decrease of the sural nerve action potentials on both sides: 2μV (normal >10μV). Nerve conduction velocity was 29m/s. The superficial peroneal nerve action potential was absent.

Blood pressure was measured at 130/70mm Hg with a heart rate of 74/minute. Upon standing, blood pressure fell to 70/40mm Hg, with a pulse rate at 70/minute and some dizziness. Electrocardiography identified a left bundle branch block and echocardiography showed a hypertrophic restrictive cardiomyopathy with an ejection fraction of 53% and an interventricular septum measurement of 14mm. A restrictive cardiomyopathy with increased thickness of the septum is highly suggestive of amyloid cardiomyopathy.

Continued overleaf

Late-onset transthyretin familial amyloid polyneuropathy *continued*

Routine blood tests including protein immunoelectrophoresis were normal. A salivary gland biopsy was normal.

The diagnosis of a late-onset, sporadic form of transthyretin familial amyloid polyneuropathy was suspected. A nerve biopsy showed amyloid deposits and DNA testing showed a *TTR-Val30Met* mutation. The patient subsequently underwent an orthotopic liver transplantation and was in a stable condition 3 years later.

Muscle strength and tendon reflexes are normal. This neurological defect typically points to the involvement of unmyelinated and small myelinated fibres.

A few months later sensory loss extends above the ankle level on both sides, with a disturbed light touch perception distally but dissociated sensory loss still present more proximally. The neurological deficit progresses relentlessly, with an extension of sensory loss towards the proximal lower limbs. Motor deficit appears in the distal lower limbs along with impairment of light touch and deep sensation, in relation to the involvement of larger sensory and motor nerve fibres. Walking becomes increasingly difficult with a loss of balance and stepping gait. Neuropathic pains are often of the burning type, worse at night and associated with allodynia.

During the following months and years sensory deficit extends to the thighs, then affects the fingers and the forearm gradually, as the anterior trunk is involved. Motor deficit also follows a length-dependent progression and walking without aid becomes increasingly difficult. Life-threatening autonomic dysfunction is present at this stage along with loss of weight and muscle wasting. Loss of pain sensation with preservation of normal or subnormal strength allows painless trauma and the development of plantar ulcers and foot osteoarthropathy (Charcot's joints). In a variable proportion of patients, however, light touch is affected early but proprioception is spared in most cases.

Late-onset FAP

In patients over 50 years of age with the *TTR-Val30Met* mutation, scattered outside the endemic areas in Japan, there is a 10/1 male preponderance. The most common initial symptom is paraesthesias in the legs, with mild symptoms of autonomic dysfunction, frequent cardiac involvement, low penetrance, and a family history in only one third of patients. Due to the late onset and low penetrance of *TTR* mutations in some areas, TTR-FAP may present as sporadic cases.

Focal manifestations at onset

Amyloid deposits may accumulate locally and induce a focal deficit of a cranial nerve, a nerve trunk or a plexus. Carpal tunnel syndrome is a common and early but non-specific manifestation of TTR-FAP.

Autonomic dysfunction

Autonomic neuropathy is nearly constant from the very beginning in early-onset TTR-FAP. Cardio-circulatory, gastrointestinal and genitourinary systems are commonly affected in this setting. They seldom precede the sensory-motor manifestations, except for intracardiac conduction failures. Cardio-circulatory dysautonomia is responsible for orthostatic hypotension, which may remain silent or cause fatigue, blurred vision or dizziness when standing up. Gastrointestinal manifestations include episodic postprandial diarrhoea, severe constipation or both alternately. Gastroparesis and postprandial vomiting cause dehydration and increase postural hypotension and progressive loss of weight. In men, erectile dysfunction is an early feature that may precede sensory symptoms of neuropathy. Autonomic dysfunction is less prominent in late-onset TTR-FAP.

Extra-neurological manifestations

Cardiac involvement is observed in 80% of cases of TTR-FAP. Progressive amyloid deposition may induce restrictive cardiomyopathy, episodes of arrhythmias and severe conduction disorders. Atrioventricular block and bundle branch blocks are common and often require implantation of a pacemaker. Cardiomyopathy seems more common among men with a non-*TTR-Val30Met* mutation and a late onset.

Vitreous opacities may cause gradual visual loss, and trabecular obstruction responsible for chronic open-angle glaucoma. Renal involvement is relatively rare. Loss of more than 10% body weight can be an early manifestation of TTR-FAP. Cachexia is inescapable after a few years. Patients become bedridden, exposed to bedsores, venous thrombosis and pulmonary embolism.

Clinical work-up

Temperature, light touch, position and vibratory senses, and pain sensation must be tested, as well as muscle strength and tendon reflexes. Motor deficit must be graded and sensory changes recorded on a chart for comparison.

Sensory action potentials, which are relatively spared in small fibre neuropathies, are often at the lower limit of normal values initially, but then gradually decrease with progression of the deficit. Quantitative sensory testing and sympathic skin tests can confirm small fibre involvement before alteration of sensory action potentials detected by routine conduction studies.

Diagnosis and diagnostic criteria

The diagnosis of TTR-FAP rests on the association of a sensory-motor and autonomic polyneuropathy with a family history for neuropathy. Demonstration of amyloid deposits in tissue biopsy is not mandatory in patients with a positive family history but confirmation by DNA testing is required.

In patients without a known family history of amyloidosis, TTR-FAP should be considered in cases with a progressive axonal polyneuropathy of unknown origin, especially when associated with autonomic dysfunction, cardiac manifestations or carpal tunnel syndrome.

A biopsy of an affected organ, especially a nerve biopsy, should then be considered, to demonstrate the presence of extracellular amyloid deposits in the endoneurial space. Amyloid deposits can also be visualised in muscle specimens, salivary glands or in abdominal fat. It must be remembered, however, that negative biopsy findings do not rule out amyloidosis. An affinity for congo red or thioflavin T staining along with a characteristic yellow-green birefringence under polarized light confirms its amyloid nature but not the type of amyloid (Figure 8). Electron microscopy examination shows the fibrillar aspect of the amyloid substance, made up of unbranched fibrils of 10nm diameter with parallel dense borders. Immunolabelling with anti-TTR antibody strongly favours the genetic origin of the disease, but DNA testing remains mandatory.

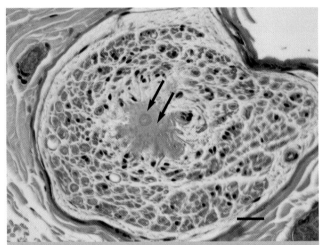

Figure 8. Familial amyloid polyneuropathy. Cross-section of a paraffin-embedded nerve biopsy specimen from a patient with familial amyloid polyneuropathy. Congo red staining shows congophilic deposits in the endoneurium of this nerve fascicle (arrows). (Bar: 20μm.)

Genetics

As of today, 119 point mutations, including 113 amyloidogenic mutations in the *TTR* gene, have been identified. Pathogenic mutations mainly cause neuropathy but some variants are associated with a predominant or isolated cardiomyopathy termed familial amyloid cardiomyopathy.

TTR-Val30Met is the most frequent substitution, resulting in a guanine to cytosine mutation in exon 2 of the gene. It is virtually the only variant detected in Portugal, Brazil and Sweden. By contrast, as many as 30 different *TTR* variants are reported in Japan and in France. A less severe phenotype occurs in patients carrying compound heterozygous mutations, which may enhance the stability of TTR tetramers.

Striking differences are observed in the expression of the disease. At age 50 years, 60% of Portuguese carriers are symptomatic (i.e. penetrance 60%), whereas it is only 18% and 11% in French and Swedish families, respectively. Genetic information can be delivered to at-risk family members. DNA testing offers the possibility of a presymptomatic predictive diagnosis. These tests are performed according to guidelines similar to those applied for other autosomal dominant neurodegenerative diseases. They require psychological support keeping in mind the late onset in some families and the variable and incomplete penetrance.

Treatment of TTR-FAP

Treatment of symptoms

Neuropathic pain is often disturbing in TTR-FAP. Gabapentin, pregabalin or duloxetine can be useful in this setting. Postural hypotension often requires the careful use of 9-alpha-fluorohydrocortisone. Implantation of a permanent pacemaker is required in most patients. Arrhythmias should be treated with antiarrhythmic drugs with or without an implantable cardioverter-defibrillator.

Control of amyloid deposits

Liver transplantation

Liver transplantation (LT) aims to prevent the formation of additional amyloid deposits by removing the liver, which is the main source of mutant TTR. A benefit of LT has been demonstrated for patients with the *TTR-Val30Met* mutation, who often survive more than 20 years these days, but LT does not prevent the development of heart arrhythmias. LT must be performed early in the course of TTR-FAP. Over 90% of patients with a pure sensory neuropathy remain stable after LT although no significant objective improvement of amyloid neuropathy occurs. The main prognostic factor after LT is the occurrence or worsening of cardiac dysfunction.

TTR stabilizers

Tafamidis and diflunisal are two well-tolerated drugs which contribute to stabilisation of the TTR tetramer and prevent further deposition of amyloid. Although they do not stop progression of TTR-FAP completely, their effect is of interest.

Gene therapy

Gene therapy is currently undergoing studies with small interfering RNAs and antisense oligonucleotides.

Apolipoprotein A1 amyloidosis

Apolipoprotein A1 amyloidosis is very rare. It is characterised by polysystemic manifestations with the age of onset in the fourth decade of life. The disease predominantly affects the kidney, liver and gastrointestinal tract. A length-dependent polyneuropathy occurs but is not a prominent feature of the disease. Progression of renal lesions can lead to chronic renal failure, dialysis, and related polyneuropathy.

Gelsolin amyloidosis

Hereditary gelsolin amyloidosis (HGA) is an autosomal dominant systemic amyloidosis, first described in 1969 in Finland. HGA is characterised by an adult onset of a slowly progressive peripheral neuropathy, with corneal lattice dystrophy, cranial neuropathy, and cutis laxa. The amyloid fibrils are composed of fragments of gelsolin generating AGel caused by a mutation of the gelsolin gene. The neuropathy is relatively mild. Only a few cases have been reported outside Finland.

Fabry's disease

Fabry disease is an X-linked lysosomal storage disorder caused by the deficient activity of the lysosomal glycohydrolase enzyme, α-galactosidase A [11]. This enzyme defect leads to the progressive accumulation of globotriaosylceramide (GL-3) and related glycosphingolipids, within vascular endothelial cells, dorsal root ganglia neuronal cells and perineurial cells (Figure 9). This neuropathy is associated with pain and decreased thermal sensation, particularly to cold, with relative preservation of large fibre function, such as vibration detection. With age, the incidence of life-threatening complications involving the kidney, heart, and brain, progresses. Strokes and transient ischaemic attacks are common. According to the Fabry Registry, the average life expectancy of men with Fabry disease is 58.2 years and that of women 75.4 years [12]. Enzyme replacement therapy has a positive effect on renal and cardiac function (especially in the early stage), gastrointestinal disturbance, neuropathic pain, thermal sensation, and sweat function.

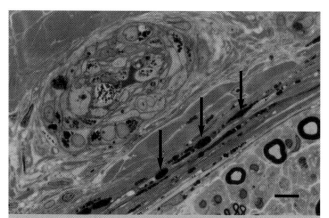

Figure 9. Fabry's disease. Cross-section of a one-micron-thick plastic-embedded nerve specimen to show characteristic osmiophilic inclusions in perineurial cells (arrows). (Bar: 10μm.)

Hereditary neuropathy with central nervous system involvement: giant axonal neuropathy

Giant axonal neuropathy (GAN) is a rare hereditary autosomal recessive neurodegenerative disease affecting both the peripheral and the central nervous system [13]. The onset occurs during the first decade of life on average. The main manifestations are peripheral sensory motor neuropathy associated with a secondary and various involvement of the central nervous system, and tightly-curled hair. It has a varying course from case to case with a diverse prognosis. On nerve biopsy all patients share the presence of a variable number of giant axons filled with neurofilament in the nerve biopsy, which represents the pathological hallmark of the disease (Figure 10). GAN is caused by mutations in the gene, *GAN*, encoding the gigaxonin protein. The disability progresses slowly. Patients become wheelchair-bound at an age that can vary between the second to the fourth decade; death occurs between the ages of 20 and 60 years.

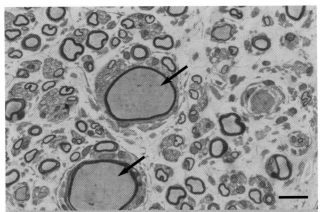

Figure 10. Giant axonal neuropathy. One-micron-thick cross-section of a plastic-embedded nerve specimen to show characteristic 'giant' axons (arrows) surrounded by a thin myelin sheath. (Thionin blue staining. Bar: 20μm.)

Hereditary neuropathies and cerebellar ataxia

A sensory neuropathy, usually asymptomatic, is present in Friedreich's disease which is mainly characterised by a severe progressive ataxia, areflexia and frequent cardiac involvement. In several other hereditary cerebellar ataxias there is a subclinical involvement of the peripheral nervous system.

In summary for this chapter, familial neuropathies account for an important proportion of chronic neuropathies, which, in addition to the burden of the disease, carry the risk of transmission of the disease to offspring. The main manifestations and features which should alert the patient and practitioners include a positive family history for neuropathy which is found in most patients with an autosomal dominant disorder. The association of neurological manifestations with skeletal abnormalities should also ring a bell. Disorders with a recessive transmission should be suspected in cases of consanguinity. When a familial neuropathy is suspected or diagnosed, the patient should be referred to an expert centre for the best management and genetic counselling.

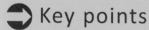 Key points

- The typical CMT phenotype is characterised by onset in the first decades of life, of slowly progressive bilateral muscle wasting and weakness starting with the feet and legs, and then gradually ascending to the distal third of the thigh and hands. It is often associated with pes cavus.

- The autosomal dominant CMT, CMT1A, is related to duplication of the 17p peripheral myelin protein 22 (*PMP22*), or less often to *PMP22* point mutation. CMT1B is related to mutation of the myelin P zero protein.

- Autosomal recessive cases are frequent in populations with a high rate of consanguineous marriages. Onset is in the first decade of life and the progression is rapid and severe.

- Hereditary sensory neuropathies encompass a variety of purely or predominantly sensory polyneuropathies that may or may not be associated with manifestations of dysautonomia.

- Hereditary neuropathies with polysystemic manifestations include autosomal dominant familial amyloid polyneuropathies (FAP) and X-linked Fabry's disease. Early liver transplantation is the first-line treatment in transthyretin-FAP.

- Genetic counselling is mandatory in these diseases.

References

1. Pareyson D, Marchesi C, Salsano E. Dominant Charcot-Marie-Tooth syndrome and cognate disorders. *Handb Clin Neurol* 2013; 115: 817-45.

2. Li J, Krajewski K, Shy ME, *et al*. Hereditary neuropathy with liability to pressure palsy: the electrophysiology fits the name. *Neurology* 2002; 58: 1769-73.

3. Parman Y, Battaloglu E. Recessively transmitted predominantly motor neuropathies. *Handb Clin Neurol* 2013; 115: 847-61.

4. Murphy SM, Laurá M, Fawcett K, *et al*. Charcot-Marie-Tooth disease: frequency of genetic subtypes and guidelines for genetic testing. *J Neurol Neurosurg Psychiatry* 2012; 83: 706-10.

5. Murphy SM, Laurá M, Reilly MM. DNA testing in hereditary neuropathies. *Handb Clin Neurol* 2013; 115: 213-32.

6. Auer-Grumbach M. Hereditary sensory and autonomic neuropathies. *Handb Clin Neurol* 2013; 115: 893-906.

7. Axelrod FB. Familial dysautonomia. *Muscle Nerve* 2004; 29: 352-63.

8. Planté-Bordeneuve V, Said G. Familial amyloid polyneuropathy. *Lancet Neurol* 2011; 10: 1086-97.

9. Ando Y, Coelho T, Berk JL. Guideline of transthyretin-related hereditary amyloidosis for clinicians. *Orphanet J Rare Dis* 2013; 20: 8-31.

10. Plante-Bordeneuve V. Update in the diagnosis and management of transthyretin familial amyloid polyneuropathy. *J Neurol* 2014; 261: 1227-33.

11. Toyooka K. Fabry disease. *Handb Clin Neurol* 2013; 115: 629-42.

12. Eng CM, Fletcher J, Wilcox WR, *et al*. Fabry disease: baseline medical characteristics of a cohort of 1765 males and females in the Fabry Registry. *J Inherit Metab Dis* 2007; 30: 184-92.

13. Hentati F, Hentati E, Amouri R. Giant axonal neuropathy. *Handb Clin Neurol* 2013; 115: 933-8.

Chapter 11

Neuropathic pain

Overview

This chapter defines the different patterns of neuropathic pain, the associated conditions and treatments available. Focal pain occurs in trigeminal neuralgia, *Herpes zoster* infection, brachial neuritis, sciatica and proximal diabetic neuropathy. Pain in generalised, length-dependent polyneuropathies is common in small fibre diabetic neuropathy. In multifocal neuropathy, pain occurs in demyelinating and axonal processes. First-line treatment includes the use of antidepressant and antiepileptic drugs. Topical treatment is used in post-herpetic neuralgia. The practical management of patients with painful neuropathy is also presented.

Introduction

Pain is the most common and disturbing symptom of peripheral neuropathy. Spontaneous pain can be the presenting symptom or complicate the course of virtually any neuropathy, yet it occurs more frequently in some neuropathies. Another type of pain, called causalgia or allodynia, which applies to the painful perception of normally non-painful stimuli, occurs frequently as a secondary phenomenon after nerve damage. In this chapter we will consider the most common causes of neuropathic pain and the management of patients with painful neuropathies.

Frequency of pain in the different patterns of neuropathy

Pain is a major component of symptoms that contribute to alter the quality of life in patients suffering from different patterns of neuropathy. The incidence of pain varies between neuropathies, but virtually all acquired neuropathies can be painful, while only a small proportion of patients with hereditary neuropathies complain of pain.

Different types of pain

Neuropathic pain characteristics vary according to the quality of pain, distribution and associated manifestations. Neuralgia applies to pain in the distribution of a nerve trunk. It can be paroxysmal or permanent, burning, or shooting in nature, the best example being trigeminal neuralgia. Allodynia applies to pain due to a stimulus that does not normally provoke pain. An example would be the unpleasant sensation caused by touching a sunburned area. Causalgia is characterised by sustained burning pain, allodynia and hyperpathia after a traumatic nerve lesion, often associated with vasomotor dysfunction in the nerve territory. When pain occurs in an anaesthetic area it is called anaesthesia dolorosa. Dysaesthesia is an unpleasant sensation, not always painful, usually provoked by a non-painful stimulus. Conversely, paraesthesia applies to a non-painful spontaneous or evoked abnormal sensation. The increased sensitivity and reaction to a non-painful stimulus is called hyperaesthesia if the stimulus is non-painful; hyperalgesia when the stimulus is painful. Hyperpathia is a painful syndrome in response to a painful stimulus.

The course of the painful syndrome is important to consider. Pain can be acute, as in sciatica or brachial neuritis. Pain lasting more than 3-6 months is called chronic, such as in post-herpetic neuralgia, in causalgia secondary to a lesion of a nerve trunk or in distal painful neuropathy. With chronic pain it is important to take into account the influence of pathophysiological, psychological and social factors in its development and persistence.

Pain in focal neuropathies

Cranial nerves: trigeminal neuralgia

Trigeminal neuralgia or 'tic douloureux de la face' stands apart in the field of painful neuropathies because pain is the only manifestation of this syndrome (⊃ see case study below). Typical trigeminal neuralgia occurs in older people, mostly after the age of 50 years. It is characterised by a one-sided, shooting, lightning-like, unbearable attack of facial pain in the territory of one of the three branches of the trigeminal nerve. This predominates in the infraorbital branch or in the lower jaw area.

Trigeminal neuralgia

Mary is a 67-year-old woman who consulted for facial pain that started 2 weeks previously. The patient was in good general condition and had no known illness. The pain was intermittent, occurring with attacks lasting a few minutes. The pain was located in the lower third of the face on the right side, in the lower jaw area. Pain was triggered by chewing, speaking and even by her face being exposed to wind. The patient stopped eating solid food to avoid chewing. She described the pain as repetitive and shooting, and tried to protect her face with her hand during these attacks, which left her exhausted. Neurological examination was normal; of note, particularly, there was no sensory or motor deficit in the third branch of the trigeminal nerve. An MRI of the brain had been performed previously, which was normal. Routine blood tests were also normal. The week before the consultation she had had two teeth removed on the same side, which did not influence the pain.

In summary, this patient had a typical trigeminal neuralgia involving the third branch of the trigeminal nerve, which is often mistaken for a dental problem.

Tegretol® 100mg three times per day was started. It was gradually increased to a total dose of 900mg/d within a couple of weeks. No disturbing side effects occurred, particularly no ataxia, and the blood cell count and sodium levels remained normal. The patient still had some minor attacks of facial pain, but these were much milder than before treatment. She will remain on treatment for an undetermined period of time.

Neurological examination is normal. There is no sensory or motor deficit. Pain occurs spontaneously or can be triggered by mechanical means, such as chewing, speaking, touching or other contact. In approximately 2% of patients, mostly younger patients, trigeminal neuralgia occurs in the setting of multiple sclerosis.

Symptomatic trigeminal neuralgia also occurs in patients with tumours and other processes of the brainstem and posterior fossa. In such cases, pain is associated with a sensory deficit in the corresponding territory and, when the third branch of the nerve is involved, with a motor deficit affecting mastication. In patients with idiopathic trigeminal neuralgia, magnetic resonance imaging (MRI) may show a neurovascular contact at the root entry zone of the nerve; however, this is also observed in 25% of asymptomatic controls.

The most common choice of drug is carbamazepine (Tegretol®), starting from 100mg daily with a gradual increase up to 1200 or even 1500mg daily if necessary. Adverse effects are more disabling at higher doses, especially after a rapid increase. They include dizziness, ataxia, impaired vision, drowsiness, headache, cutaneous rashes, and leucopenia. Regular blood counts, liver transaminases and blood sodium levels must be checked at the beginning of treatment and after a few weeks.

Phenytoin can be used at a dose of 300-500mg per day in association with carbamazepine.

Surgical procedures may be necessary when trigeminal neuralgia does not respond to drugs and in cases where compression of the trigeminal root by a vascular loop is seen on imaging. Percutaneous thermo-coagulation is often preferred to surgery after suboccipital craniotomy.

Herpes zoster and post-herpetic neuralgia (PHN)

Herpes zoster is a disease of the elderly and of the immunocompromised. People over 60 years of age have an 8-10-fold increased incidence of *Herpes zoster* compared with those under the age of 60. Immunocompromised individuals, including AIDS patients, have an increased disease prevalence at a younger age. The condition might be preceded by paraesthesias, itching and pain. The sensory symptoms may be severe enough to suggest a coronary ischaemia or an abdominal condition. Pain and itching are usually concomitant with the eruption, but they may precede the eruption and in the vast majority of cases improve after a few weeks. Unfortunately, chronic post-herpetic pain in the elderly is relatively common following the appearance of skin lesions.

Post-herpetic pain (PHN) is defined as pain in the distribution of the rash which persists beyond 4-6 weeks following shingles. The risk for PHN increases with age, and almost half of patients over 60 years who suffer from *Herpes zoster* will develop it, immunocompromised patients being more susceptible. The pain involves the affected dermatome and is usually severe, burning, lancinating and constant. In fact, it can be so disturbing as to lead to severe depression and even suicide.

The treatment of PHN is usually difficult and the pain in many cases may be intractable. There is no accepted regimen and agents that have been shown to possess some clinical efficacy may include: tricyclic antidepressants (amitriptyline), calcium channel α2-δ ligands (gabapentin, pregabalin), patches of topical lidocaine, opioid agonists, and anticonvulsants (sodium valproate). Topical application of capsaicin ointment, four times a day, may help.

Radicular pains

Acute or subacute radicular pain is a major symptom of brachial neuritis and in sciatica. Pain is also a major symptom of the meningoradiculoneuritis of Lyme disease (⊙ see case study on p90, Chapter 7 — Infectious neuropathies). When radicular pain is related to disc compression it is often self-limiting, lasting a few weeks or months. Radicular pain is usually well controlled by immobilisation of the spine. Occasionally surgery is needed to remove a disc herniation or a tumour.

Brachial plexus

Brachial neuritis is also an acute or subacute symptom. It is characterised by sharp, severe pain in the nerves of the brachial plexus, followed by weakness or numbness. The cause of acute brachial neuritis is unknown. The course extends over a few months in most cases. Pain responds to corticosteroids, at least partially. Residual weakness is common.

In radiation-induced brachial plexopathy, pain is less common and disturbing than in plexopathy due to invasion by malignant cells.

Proximal diabetic neuropathy

Diabetic patients usually over the age of 50, mostly with type 2 diabetes, may present with proximal neuropathy of the lower limbs characterised by a variable degree of pain and sensory loss over the anterior aspect of the thigh, associated with uni- or bilateral proximal muscle weakness and atrophy. The patient complains of numbness or pain of the anterior aspect of the thigh, often of the burning type, worse at night and associated with allodynia. Pain and proximal weakness are usually associated with insomnia and a marked loss of weight. Pain usually subsides after a few weeks or months. In cases with a protracted course and pain resisting symptomatic treatment, prescription of corticosteroids for a few weeks can induce a dramatic improvement (see Chapter 8 — Diabetic and uraemic neuropathies). An adjustment in the treatment of diabetes is usually required.

Pain in generalised polyneuropathy

Length-dependent diabetic polyneuropathy (LDDP)

Small fibre neuropathy
In this group lesions predominate on small myelinated and unmyelinated nerve fibres, accounting for the impairment of pain and temperature sensation.

Length-dependent diabetic polyneuropathy (LDDP) is the most common cause of painful neuropathy in the world. Several million people worldwide are affected by diabetic neuropathic pain. LDDP usually becomes symptomatic years after the onset of type 1, but is often the first and only manifestation of type 2 diabetes of mature onset. The initial 'positive' manifestations of sensory neuropathy include numbness, burning feet, a pins and needles sensation, and lancinating pains — often worse at night and by contact (➲ see case studies on pp120-22, Chapter 8 — Diabetic and uraemic neuropathies). Acute painful neuropathy with allodynia is sometimes associated with cachexia and depression, especially in young adults with type 1 diabetes. In a study performed in Liverpool, the prevalence of painful neuropathy was estimated to be four times more common in people with diabetes than in the control sample [1]. The prevalence of diabetic peripheral neuropathy increases with age, and tends to be more common in patients with type 2 than in those with type 1 diabetes (see Chapter 8 — Diabetic and uraemic neuropathies). The precipitation of acute painful neuropathy can also follow the establishment of tight glycaemic control. In painful LDDP, nerve biopsy shows an association of loss of nerve fibres with regeneration by axonal sprouting, which may cause spontaneous pain and allodynia by spontaneous firing [2]. In LDDP, the antioxidant, α-lipoic acid, is licensed only in some countries for the treatment of diabetic polyneuropathy and is found to improve pain [3].

Amyloid polyneuropathy is also an important cause of small fibre neuropathy, associated with a range of sensory and motor progressive length-dependent deficits to severe autonomic dysfunction. Familial and acquired, light chain, amyloid neuropathies are often associated with severe neuropathic pain, which have much the same characteristics as those observed in diabetic patients. (See Chapter 10 — Hereditary neuropathies.)

Large fibre neuropathy

In alcoholic neuropathy and in neuropathies due to malnutrition, nerve lesions markedly predominate on larger myelinated fibres. Symptoms are often marked by severe neuropathic pain with spontaneous pain and allodynia predominating on the distal lower limbs.

Acute pain, especially triggered by contact, occurs during and shortly after infusion of oxaliplatin. In 95% of patients, oxaliplatin causes an acute syndrome of severe cold hypersensitivity, jaw tightness, cramps, and perioral, pharyngeal and limb paraethesias soon after infusion which resolves within hours or days.

Thalidomide can induce a painful neuropathy in patients treated for multiple myeloma. The clinical features are those of a painful sensory length-dependent axonal neuropathy or less frequently a sensory neuronopathy. Patients present with symptoms of numbness, paraesthesias which may be painful, and cramps starting in the feet.

Non-length-dependent polyneuropathy

Demyelinating polyneuropathy

Guillain-Barré syndrome (GBS)

Pain has been mentioned in up to 50% of patients in many reports [4]. GBS pain at onset usually simulates the sensation that occurs hours or a day after strenuous exercise. Common locations are the lower back and large muscles of the thighs and buttocks, sometimes accompanied by sciatica (◔ see case study on p44, Chapter 4 — Guillain-Barré syndrome). Another pain syndrome results from intense distal paraesthesias. Pain is often worse at night. Severe muscle pain usually subsides as muscle strength improves.

Residual pain can occur 1 or 2 years after the onset of GBS, with disabling sensory symptoms having been reported in up to 15% of patients. Distal burning dysaesthesias precipitated by contact or pressure may occur in patients who have otherwise complete motor recovery. Paraesthesias may be exacerbated by exertion, heat or cold.

Subacute and chronic inflammatory demyelinating polyneuropathy (CIDP)

Pain is less common in subacute and chronic inflammatory demyelinating polyneuropathy (Figure 1). Yet in a report by Bouchard et al, 30% of patients complained of pain at the onset of the neuropathy, which extended over a month, with 8% still complaining of pain in a steady state [5].

Axonal multifocal neuropathies

Pain is an important and nearly constant component of the ischaemic neuropathy observed in vasculitis, the major cause of multifocal axonal

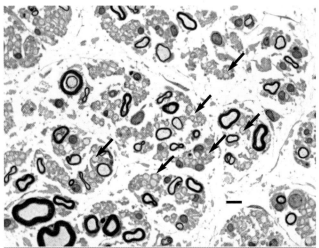

Figure 1. One-micron-thick cross-section of a plastic-embedded sural nerve biopsy specimen from a patient with painful chronic inflammatory demyelinating polyneuropathy. The density of unmyelinated fibres (arrows), or C fibres, which convey pain sensation, is normal in this case. Normal: 17,000-35,000 unmyelinated fibres per mm². (Bar: 5μm.)

neuropathy (see case study on p72, Chapter 6 — Vasculitic neuropathies). Pain occurs both as an early manifestation of ischaemic neuropathy, in which case it responds well to treatment with corticosteroids, and as a residual manifestation subsequent to axonal lesions of nerve trunks, with sensory loss and allodynia.

Management of patients with neuropathic pain [6]

Symptomatic pharmacological treatment

Neuropathic pain often requires treatment specifically for pain relief. Due to the frequency of painful diabetic neuropathies, most controlled studies have been performed in patients with distal diabetic polyneuropathy.

Antidepressants

Antidepressants have a beneficial effect on most cases of neuropathic pain.

Tricyclic antidepressants (TCAs) (amitriptyline and imipramine) and the mixed serotonin and noradrenaline reuptake inhibitors (duloxetine and venlafaxine) can be used. Response and tolerance to these drugs are very variable. In our experience small doses of amitriptyline have a favourable effect in most cases of chronic neuropathic pain. Effective doses vary considerably between patients. An associated small dose of clonazepam, such as 0.5-2mg/day, can help. Pain relief is independent of the antidepressant activity of the drug. Adverse events related to the anticholinergic actions of TCAs (e.g. dry mouth, constipation, nausea, difficulty emptying the bladder, hypotension) are common in addition to drowsiness, fatigue, and weight gain. Somnolence and gait disturbances are common in the elderly. Orthostatic hypotension is another possible side effect, especially in diabetic patients. Electrocardiography (ECG) should always be obtained prior to treatment, and TCAs should not be used in patients with cardiac conduction disturbances, cardiac failure, and epilepsy.

Duloxetine is easy to administer; the starting dose is 30mg and the dose can be increased to 60mg once daily. Venlafaxine is administered twice daily in doses up to 150-225mg daily.

Antiepileptic drugs

Many anticonvulsants have a pharmacological action that may interfere with neuronal hyperexcitability, by decreasing excitatory or increasing inhibitory transmission. This way, anticonvulsants may attenuate the neuronal hyperexcitability responsible for chronic pain conditions. Carbamazepine is mainly used with success in trigeminal neuralgia. The most common side effects of carbamazepine are sedation, dizziness, ataxia, blurred vision, hyponatremia, confusion in elderly patients, and in rare cases blood dyscrasia. The starting dose is usually 300mg daily and the dose is increased by 100mg every other day to 1500-2000mg/day.

Gabapentin and pregabalin are a new generation of anticonvulsants. The most common side effects of gabapentin and pregabalin are central nervous system-related side effects with dizziness and somnolence. Gabapentin is initiated with 300mg daily, which is slowly increased to a final daily dose of between 1800 and 3600mg, and administered three times daily. Pregabalin may be initiated with 75 or 150mg daily and increased up to 600mg in two divided doses. Dose reduction is needed in patients with impaired renal function. Patients failing to respond to one of these drugs may benefit from the other.

Opioids

Morphine and oxycodone have been shown to have an effect in painful neuropathies, although this is based on a limited number of studies. Tramadol is an opioid with a monoaminergic reuptake inhibitory action which may also relieve neuropathic pain. Before initiating treatment it is therefore important to address risk factors for abuse.

Topical treatments

A lidocaine (5%) medicated patch is indicated for the relief of pain associated with post-herpetic neuralgia, or with localised neuropathic pain. High-dose (8%) capsaicin patches are approved for the treatment of peripheral neuropathic pain and for the treatment of post-herpetic neuralgia. After treating the skin area with a local anaesthetic, the capsaicin patch remains applied for 30-60 minutes. The effect starts within 1 day to 2 weeks after the application. The treatment may be repeated every 3 months.

Non-pharmacological treatments

For patients receiving pharmacological treatment, the average pain reduction is about 20-30%, and only 20-35% of patients will achieve at least a 50% pain reduction with available drugs. Non-pharmacological treatments need to be used alongside pharmacological treatments. These treatments include physiotherapy, cognitive and behavioural therapy, and hypnosis.

Transcutaneous electrical nerve stimulation and acupuncture are sometimes used but their efficacy in painful neuropathy is not well established.

Spinal cord stimulation is a technique whereby electrodes are inserted percutaneously or during open surgery into the posterior epidural space to stimulate the dorsal column of the spinal cord to replace a painful sensation with paraesthesia [7].

Spinal cord stimulation is generally reserved for patients who have failed conservative management. Psychological clearance is generally recommended. Prior to permanent placement, the patient undergoes implantation of a trial stimulation. Pain relief of 50% or greater is generally acceptable in order to progress to permanent implantation. The trial period usually lasts between 5 and 7 days and permanent spinal cord stimulators are placed several weeks after a successful trial. Spinal cord stimulation is currently approved for chronic pain of the trunk and limbs.

Practical management of patients

Studies suggest that tricyclic antidepressants (TCAs), serotonin noradrenaline reuptake inhibitors (SNRIs), gabapentin, and pregabalin have comparable efficacy in neuropathic pain, so they tend to be the first drugs of choice.

In patients with focal peripheral neuropathy with allodynia, a topical lidocaine patch is also a first-line drug. Tricyclic antidepressants or duloxetine may be the first drug of choice in patients with depression. Combination therapy may be considered in patients with an insufficient effect from one drug.

Treatment is usually a trial-and-error process and has to be individualised to each patient, taking into account all comorbidities such as possible concomitant depression, anxiety, diseases, and drug interactions. Before choosing a neuropathic pain treatment, clinicians need to consider the benefits and possible side effects of a specific treatment.

After establishing the diagnosis of painful neuropathy, the underlying disease should be identified and treated, whenever possible. When the underlying mechanisms causing the pain cannot be treated, symptomatic treatment of pain and related disability should be offered. Realistic expectations for the outcome of a given treatment should be discussed with the patient, explaining that often only partial pain relief from neuropathic pain can be expected, and that sensory deficits are unlikely to respond to treatment.

The treatment effect is usually assessed by a reduction in pain intensity on a visual analogue scale or an 11-point numerical rating scale ranging from 'no pain' to 'worst possible pain'. This measure can be supplemented with other similar scales that assess the degree of pain relief. Various measures of quality of life can also be added. In the case of partial pain relief, another drug with complementary mechanisms can be added. There is a good rationale for combining drugs with a different mode of action because this may lower the frequency and severity of side effects and have an additive and maybe even a synergistic effect, but there is still limited clinical evidence for these assumptions. There is some evidence for combining gabapentin with an opioid or an antidepressant. Side effects may be a limiting factor and it is important to monitor the patient for additive adverse effects. Treatment to alleviate pain should be associated with treatment of the cause of the neuropathy when feasible.

Patients with refractory chronic neuropathic pain can be referred to pain management units where a multidisciplinary team with pain nurses, physiotherapists, and psychologists can handle the different aspects and consequences of chronic pain in daily activities.

⭢ Key points

- Typical trigeminal neuralgia occurs mostly after the age of 50 years. It is a one-sided, shooting, lightning-like, unbearable attack of facial pain in the territory of one of the three branches of the trigeminal nerve. There is no neurological deficit. Trigeminal neuralgia responds well to treatment with carbamazepine.

- Post-herpetic pain is chronic and extremely disabling. The local application of a lidocaine or capsaicin patch can help.

- Length-dependent diabetic polyneuropathy is the most common cause of painful neuropathy in the world.

- Tricyclic antidepressants (amitriptyline and imipramine) and the mixed serotonin and noradrenaline reuptake inhibitors (duloxetine and venlafaxine) often work.

- Many anticonvulsants (carbamazepine, gabapentin and pregabalin) are indicated in chronic neuropathic pain.

- Tramadol is an opioid with a monoaminergic reuptake inhibitory action which may also relieve neuropathic pain.

- In pain clinics a multidisciplinary team (including pain nurses, physiotherapists, and psychologists) is often involved in the treatment of neuropathic pain.

References

1.   Daousi C, MacFarlane IA, Woodward A, et al. Chronic painful peripheral neuropathy in an urban community: a controlled comparison of people with and without diabetes. Diabet Med 2004; 21: 976-82.

2.   Said G, Baudoin D, Toyooka K. Axonal regeneration, motor deficit and pains in severe length-dependent diabetic polyneuropathy. J Neurol 2008; 255: 1693-702.

3. Ziegler D, Ametov A, Barinov A, *et al*. Oral treatment with alpha-lipoic acid improves symptomatic diabetic polyneuropathy: the SYDNEY 2 trial. *Diabetes Care* 2006; 29: 2365-70.

4. Ropper AH, Wijdicks EFM, Truax BT. Guillain Barré syndrome. FA Davis Company: Philadelphia, 1991.

5. Bouchard C, Lacroix C, Planté V, *et al*. Clinico-pathological findings and prognosis of chronic inflammatory demyelinating polyneuropathy. *Neurology* 1999; 52: 498-503.

6. Review in Finnerup NB, Sindrup SH, Jensen TS. Management of painful neuropathies. *Handb Clin Neurol* 2013; 115: 279-92.

7. Song JJ, Popescu A, Bell RL. Present and potential use of spinal cord stimulation to control chronic pain. *Pain Physician* 2014; 17: 235-46.

Index

S

T